Muscular Dystrophy in Children

A Guide for Families

Muscular Dystrophy in Children

A Guide for Families

Irwin M. Siegel, M.D.

Demos

Demos Medical Publishing, Inc., 386 Park Avenue South, New York, New York 10016

Library of Congress Cataloging-in-Publication Data
Siegel, Irwin M., 1927–
   Muscular dystrophy in children : a guide for families / Irwin M.
  Siegel.
     p. cm.
  Includes bibliographical references (p.).
  ISBN 1-888799-33-1
   1. Muscular dystrophy in children Popular works. 2. Neuromuscular
diseases in children Popular works. I. Title.
  RJ482.D9S56 1999
  618.92′748—dc21   99-23878
                                             CIP

Printed in Canada

You may give them your love but not your thoughts,
For they have their own thoughts.
You may house their bodies but not their souls,
For their souls dwell in the house of tomorrow, which
you cannot visit, not even in your dreams.
You may strive to be like them, but seek not to make
them like you.
For life goes not backward nor tarries with yesterday.
You are the bows from which your children as living
arrows are sent forth.

Kahlil Gibran—*On Children*

*This book is dedicated to
David, Chani, Jane, and Susan—my children.*

The kind of life lived by a patient under conditions of vigorous response to a challenge is initially preferable to a crunching, desperate winding down.

Norman Cousins, *Human Options*

CONTENTS

ACKNOWLEDGMENTS

The author wishes to acknowledge the following for their help in the preparation of this book:

Jackie Abern, CMT, for her patient editorial assistance, transcription, and reworking of the manuscript.

Patricia Casey, MS, OTR/L for her expert proofreading and critical comments.

Syed Maghrabi for bibliographical assistance; Bridget Carey, Patient Service Coordinator, MDA, for her review of the material and valuable suggestions.

Margaret Wahl, Senior Medical and Science Writer, MDA, for her critical review and helpful suggestions.

The clinic staff of the Muscle Disease Clinics of the Rush-Presbyterian–St.Luke's Medical Center and the Evanston Hospital for their able help with the multidisciplined management of our patient roster.

Chris Galietta and Mike Fitzhenry, Seating Consultants, Metro Rehab, Worth, Illinois, for keeping our patients comfortable and functional in their wheelchairs and for keeping me up to date on the latest in mobility technology.

Orthotist Gene Bernardoni and his able staff at the Ballert Orthotic Laboratory, Chicago, Illinois, and Ron Grimaud, Scheck & Siress, Inc., Chicago, Illinois, for assistance in their area of expertise.

My able colleagues, Drs. Matthew Meriggioli, Judd Jensen, Robert Wright, Peter Heydemann, Larry Bernstein, Nicholas Vick, and the late Dr. Harold L. Klawans, for continuing tuition in the fascinating fields of myology, neuromuscular disease, and allied neurologic conditions.

The Muscular Dystrophy Association, particularly Robert Ross, Senior Vice President and Executive Director, for his encouragement and support.

Demos Medical Publishing, Inc., of New York, especially Diana M. Schneider, Ph.D., Publisher, and Joan Wolk, Managing Editor, for patiently and skill-fully shepherding the book through editing and publication.

FOREWORD

My tenure with the Muscular Dystrophy Association is now nearly half a century long, and my friendship with Dr. Irwin Siegel spans nearly all of it. In that time I have known celebrities, physicians, scientists, and families affected by muscular dystrophy by the score. It would be hard to bring to mind anyone who combines better the knowledge and skills of a physician and surgeon with a parent's perspective and a gentleman's manner than does Irwin Siegel.

This book, the latest in a series of many he has authored, reflects the extraordinary qualities of this long-time MDA clinic director and current MDA vice president. Two of Dr. Siegel's previous works, published and distributed nationwide in both English and Spanish versions by MDA, have long been key elements of our publications armamentarium.

When I first received the manuscript of *Muscular Dystrophy in Children: A Guide for Families*, I found I could not put it down and ended up staying up late for a couple of nights reading it and imagining how it would help the parents who are its intended audience.

This book, which complements MDA's recent publication on the same subject, *Journey of Love* (for parents of children with the Duchenne form of muscular dystrophy), will be a great comfort and guide for those coping with the challenges of raising a child with an uncertain future. It covers everything from available medical treatments to helping the child grow up with a positive self-image to what the future holds for the treatment of muscular dystrophy—and more.

MDA's mission is to provide not only hope for a cure for muscular dystrophy, but also help, in the form of information and services that both instruct and reassure. This book provides these crucial benefits.

Robert Ross
Senior Vice President and Executive Director
Muscular Dystrophy Association
January 1999

PREFACE

If you are reading this book, you probably have or are related to a child with muscular dystrophy, or know of a family faced with this serious medical problem. This guide offers information and practical advice on the disease and its management.

The fact that some children have muscular dystrophy while others are healthy is indeed unfair. You are not the first person who will be faced with the problems of dealing with this situation, and unfortunately you won't be the last.

This book was written with you in mind. It was written for children with muscle disease, their parents, families, and other caregivers. This includes siblings, teachers, and friends. It was written because of a perceived and expressed need to guide the patient and his/her caregivers through the often frightening labyrinth of medical care that one enters when given the diagnosis of muscular dystrophy. The book will help you understand the significance of the signs and symptoms of muscular dystrophy, the treatment options available, prognosis (forecast of the probable course or outcome of a disease and what may affect it), the choices you have in directing therapy, and the trend of current research into neuromuscular diseases. However, it is not to be regarded as specific medical advice. You should always consult with your doctor regarding matters of diagnosis and treatment.

The book is construed to inform and educate with state-of-the-art information. Its goal is to address your questions and concerns in the most forthright and honest manner possible and to clearly define the available medical options at every stage of the disease and offer you guidance even when it may seem that nothing can be done.

1

INTRODUCTION

It has been said that "incurable is not untreatable."
That is the thesis of this book in a nutshell. At least
for now (and this should change), there is no cure for
muscular dystrophy. However, numerous therapies
are available to add life to a patient's years and even
years to his or her life. In some instances this includes
medication; in others hands-on manual treatments.
Surgery and bracing may play a role. The separate
and combined skills of many health professionals are
brought to bear on the multifaceted problems of the
person with a neuromuscular disease. New diagnostic
methods—many of which rely on the evolving field of
molecular genetics—ensure accurate and early diagnosis. A program of multidisciplined aggressive therapy guarantees the best treatments available.

This book examines muscular dystrophy and
related neuromuscular diseases. It takes you through
each stage in the evolution of the disease from diagno-

sis through early childhood, puberty, adolescence, and adulthood. For each of these periods we consider treatment and prognosis, problems and concerns. What is most important to me is what worries you. We will talk about these things. The text has been designed to be both pertinent and practical. It has been drawn from countless queries from numerous persons over many years and reviewed by many patients, parents, and other caregivers, as well as health professionals who work in the field of neuromuscular disease. Their suggestions have been incorporated in the book. Emphasis has been placed on crises that may arise, emotional as well as physical.

When considering muscular dystrophy, "the family is the patient." Because this is always the case, we look at the patient in the home, the community, and his or her educational setting. You will be given information on adapting to the evolving needs of the person with muscular dystrophy, sources for support, and suggestions for further reading. Tough questions will be asked and answered.

The diagnosis of muscular dystrophy can be devastating. However, the possibility of discovering a cure through energetic ongoing worldwide research is better now than it ever was. In the meanwhile children with these diseases require management. The Muscular Dystrophy Association (MDA) is a not-for-profit volunteer health agency. Since its founding in 1950, it has provided comprehensive medical services to tens of thousands of people with neuromuscular disease at more than 200 hospital-affiliated clinics across America. The association's worldwide research program funds some 400 individual scientific investigations annually. It represents the largest single effort to advance the knowledge of neuromuscular diseases and to find cures and treatments for them. The Muscular Dystrophy Association underwrites 150 chapters in the United States and Puerto Rico, providing many direct services. These include diagnosis and follow-up care from specialists in neuromuscular disease in its clinics, as well as assistance with the purchase and repair of wheelchairs and orthoses, recreation at MDA-sponsored summer camps, and select transportation assistance.

The Muscular Dystrophy Association is seeking the causes of and cures and treatments for 40 neuromuscular disorders. Its scientists are in the forefront of gene therapy research and currently are testing potential treatments for several neuromuscular diseases. Funded almost entirely by volunteer contributions from concerned individuals and cooperating organizations, the MDA conducts far-reaching educational programs for the public and medical professionals. The organization distributes a wide variety of printed and audiovisual materials to foster public understanding of neuromuscular disease. To increase knowledge of these diseases among medical professionals, the MDA sponsors scientific symposia and other meetings of neuromuscular specialists.

Information about the MDA's clinical services and research may be obtained by contacting the Muscular Dystrophy Association, National Headquarters, 3300 East Sunrise Drive, Tucson AZ 85718-3208, phone (520) 529-2000, or WWW.MDAUSA.ORG.

2

CHILDHOOD MUSCULAR DYSTROPHY

Many muscle-wasting diseases are caused by genetic defects that lead to an aberrant or absent muscle protein. Most of these proteins function to lend support to the muscle fiber but some are active in the metabolism of the cell. *Muscular dystrophy* (muscle—faulty nutrition) refers to a group of genetic diseases that are characterized by progressive weakness caused by degeneration of voluntary muscle. Cardiac and even smooth muscle also may be affected in some types of muscular dystrophy. A few forms involve other organ systems as well.

The muscular dystrophies affect an estimated 200,000 Americans; approximately two thirds of them are children. The major types of muscular dystrophy found in children are Duchenne, Becker, limb-girdle, facioscapulohumeral, congenital, myotonic, and Emery-Dreifuss muscular dystrophy. All these diseases are caused by genetic defects. Duchenne and

Becker dystrophies represent a single disease with a variation in severity. Although a family history of the disease usually is present, a sporadic mutation may cause an isolated case in any family without a history of inheritance.

HEREDITY

There are three main forms of inheritance through which muscular dystrophy can be passed from a parent to a child. These are *autosomal recessive, autosomal dominant,* and *X-linked recessive* (Figure 2-1). Inheritance by an autosomal dominant pattern occurs when only one parent needs to pass on a defective gene in order for a condition to be expressed. The offspring have a 50 percent (one in two) risk of inheriting an autosomal dominant disease. When *both* parents must pass on defective genes in order for a disease to occur, the child can inherit a *recessive* disease. Children of parents who carry a gene from the same recessive disease therefore run a 25 percent (one in four) risk of inheritance. If one gene in the pair is defective and the other gene is normal, the child becomes a *carrier* and will have minimal, if any, symptoms or signs of the disease.

Defects on the X chromosome, which determines a child's sex, lead to *X-linked* disease. These disorders (which include Duchenne muscular dystrophy, hemophilia, and red-green color blindness) are passed exclusively by the female to the male. This is because males have only one X chromosome with a Y chromosome instead of a second X chromosome in reserve, whereas females have two X chromosomes. Every son born to a female carrier of an X-linked disease (such

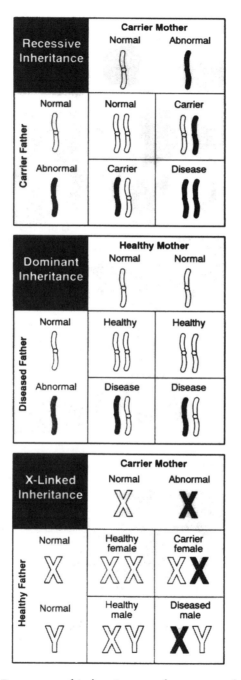

FIGURE 2–1 Patterns of inheritance for muscular dystrophy.

as hemophilia or Duchenne muscular dystrophy) runs a 50 percent risk of inheriting the abnormal gene. Each daughter has a 50 percent chance of becoming a carrier.

DUCHENNE MUSCULAR DYSTROPHY

Duchenne muscular dystrophy (DMD) is the most common childhood form of muscular dystrophy. To arrive at this diagnosis, your doctor may have to rule out other neuromuscular diseases. These include polymyositis or dermatomyositis, both of which are inflammatory muscle diseases characterized by listlessness, severe malaise (discomfort), weakness, and skin rash in the case of dermatomyositis. Other diseases that must be considered are the childhood form of facioscapulohumeral muscular dystrophy, which primarily involves the face and shoulders; congenital muscular dystrophy, a group of muscular diseases found at birth; Emery-Dreifuss muscular dystrophy, an X-linked recessive disease characterized by severe contractures and cardiac abnormalities; and neonatal myotonic dystrophy, presenting symptoms of which include profound weakness, club feet, typical facial expression, and the onset of myotonia (excessive muscle contraction on stimulation) later in its course. The signs, symptoms, and course of Becker muscular dystrophy are similar to those of Duchenne dystrophy but generally appear later and progress slower.

The differential diagnosis of Duchenne dystrophy also includes diseases of nerve, particularly a loss of motor nerve cells in the spinal cord leading to severe weakness called spinal muscular atrophy (SMA).

Duchenne dystrophy is an X-linked disease that is carried by the mother and affects only her sons. Non-hereditary cases (approximately one third of all reported cases) also occur. Children with the disease may walk late (at 18 months on average) but there is no correlation between late walking and severity or rapid progression of the disease. Early signs are evident at approximately age 4 years and include falling, difficulty getting up, difficulty ascending stairs, and a waddling broad-based gait that is the result of symmetric weakness of the muscles of the shoulders, back, hips, and legs. As the disease advances there is an increase in lumbar lordosis (swayback) as the child tries to balance himself over his weakened legs. The calves are enlarged because of initial work hypertrophy (overgrowth) followed by degeneration and the substitution of fat for muscle.

The defect in Duchenne muscular dystrophy is an absence of the muscle protein *dystrophin,* which apparently contributes to the mechanical integrity of the cell membrane of the muscle fiber. Dystrophin also is present in involuntary (smooth) muscle, as well as in the brain, heart, and retina in the back of the eyes. Although dystrophin represents only 0.002 percent of total muscle protein, its absence is devastating to muscular function. Mild nonprogressive mental retardation accompanies the disease in a small number of children. There are no abnormalities of the sphincter muscles that control bowel and bladder function. Cardiomyopathy—muscular dystrophy of the heart muscle—occurs late in the course of Duchenne muscular dystrophy, as does respiratory difficulty, usually well after a wheelchair is needed.

Diagnosis is made on the basis of a typical history and clinical presentation; a substantial elevation of creatine phosphokinase (CK), a muscle enzyme that accelerates an energy-producing chemical reaction and is elevated in muscle disease (as high as 50 to 100 times normal); a typical pattern on electromyography (EMG); DNA studies revealing an absence or abnormality of the dystrophin gene; and/or a muscle biopsy that shows typical histologic (tissue) features and lack of dystrophin by immunochemical staining.

The average age of diagnosis of DMD ranges from 4.5 to 5.5 years. Approximately 15 percent of all DMD patients are born as "secondary" cases, with parents unaware of the presence of the disease in an older child. As soon as a diagnosis of DMD is made, it becomes important to counsel mothers and female siblings about the risk of pregnancy. Mothers of an affected son who also have an affected brother, maternal uncle, sister's son, or other dystrophic male relatives in the female line of inheritance are considered *definite carriers*. Such a mother may also have affected sons by nonconsanguineous fathers. *Probable carriers* are mothers of two or more sons with muscular dystrophy who have no other affected relatives. Mothers of isolated cases and sisters and other female relatives of affected males are considered *possible carriers*. They may have a *known* risk (e.g., the daughter of a definite carrier, where the risk is 50 percent) or an unknown risk (e.g., the sister of a sporadic case).

Carriers may exhibit mild physical findings such as limb-girdle (shoulder and hip) muscle weakness and/or cramping and calf enlargement (often only on one side). Such symptoms and signs are found in approximately 8 percent of carriers. Heart problems are not uncommon in DMD carriers. Sometimes a carrier may have more severe involvement that causes weakness similar to a boy with DMD. Such is the "manifesting carrier." Scattered abnormal (myopathic) changes may be seen on EMG as well as changes on muscle biopsy, including deficiency of dystrophin. Creatine phosphokinase is increased in approximately 70 percent of carriers, with a much higher detection rate in childhood. There also is a blood test to compare a suspected carrier's DNA with that of her involved brother. Occasionally a woman will carry the genetic mutation only in some of her egg cells, which makes it difficult to test for the carrier state.

The sex of a fetus can be determined by amniocentesis at 16 to 20 weeks of pregnancy. Given the prognosis of the disorder, the pregnancy may be terminated, if desired, if the fetus is a male in a proven carrier. Prenatal diagnosis of muscular dystrophy in the fetus can be made at some medical centers by DNA analysis of cells taken from the amniotic fluid. Risks of amniocentesis include a 1:1000 rate of infection and a 1:200 incidence of spontaneous abortion. First-trimester fetal sexing is possible with a chorionic (fetal membrane) biopsy. This procedure also is useful for DNA studies of the fetus to establish a prenatal diagnosis of DMD.

The diagnosis of Duchenne muscular dystrophy presents a psychological crisis. Great emotional stress is placed on the family at this time. Guilt often is felt by and projected to the mother because of the X-linked nature of genetic transmission. Of course, responsibility should be shared between both father and mother if for no other reason than the fact that the father's chromosomes determine the sex of the child. Realistic but hopeful feedback (not pity) is required if the child is to develop a capacity for durable interpersonal relationships and an ability to establish the meaningful and stable identity that leads to self-acceptance.

The family dealing with a disabled child need not necessarily become a disabled family. Group therapy has proved valuable in assisting parents of children with neuromuscular disease by helping them develop insight and increasing communication through sharing of experiences. Access to such groups often is available through your local MDA chapter.

At the time of diagnosis, age 4 to 5 years, your child may seem hardly disabled at all. He may be a little clumsy and you might notice that he has trouble keeping up with playmates in running games. He may tire a little more easily than other children his age, and he might even complain of some cramping in his legs with strenuous activity. There is no need for special attention at this time. Every effort should be made to mainstream him in both the community and the preschool settings. He should be treated as a child first, and only afterward as a child with muscle disease. Networking with other families who are raising a child with muscular dystrophy may be useful for sharing experiences and day-to-day problem solving. The Muscular Dystrophy Association can provide you with a networking list of such families.

Although there is no need for specific occupational therapy (OT) or physical therapy (PT) at this stage, it is important to avoid prolonged bedrest. Muscle strength is lost at 3 percent to 5 percent a day at complete bedrest. Because of this, the average childhood illness should be managed by encouraging the child to stand and walk around the house as much as possible. Only life-threatening conditions warrant full bedrest.

You undoubtedly will have many questions about muscular dystrophy in general and your child in particular. Your doctor should be able to answer these questions for you. You also are encouraged to use the MDA website, which accesses experts in the field worldwide (WWW.MDAUSA.ORG) for answers to any particular questions or concerns. Here are a few of the many questions that you may have.

QUESTIONS

Q: Is it worthwhile to seek a second opinion on the diagnosis of muscular dystrophy?

A: It can't hurt, and as long as you are not wasting your time and money shopping all over the country for a better diagnosis, seeking a specialist and relying on his or her expertise should dispel any concern that your case has been misdiagnosed.

Q: How much should I tell my other children?

A: Keeping "deep dark secrets" is no way to foster healthy intrafamily relationships. Normal siblings often feel either responsible for their diseased sibling or guilty about their own normality. Children should be reassured that they were not responsible and informed at a level they can understand that their brother or sister has a weakening condition that will require patient understanding and assistance. The normal sibling can be engaged to provide some of this.

Q: Why does the young child with muscular dystrophy often have flat feet?

A: Because he has tight heel cords that prevent flexing the ankle up (dorsiflexing) during walking. Instead he must flatten his arch and roll over his foot when walking.

Q: Does Duchenne muscular dystrophy affect any particular race more than any other? Is it contagious?

A: Duchenne muscular dystrophy does not discriminate. All races are affected equally. Like other neuromuscular diseases, it is not contagious.

Q: Can my child receive immunizations?

A: The child with muscular dystrophy should be immunized just like any other child. This includes not only DPT but also flu vaccines and Pneumovax.

Q: Should I restrict the activity of my child with DMD?

A: Not at all! Children with muscle disease should be encouraged to participate in physical activities as much as possible. A child is not overactive if he is well rested after a night's sleep. Children should not be encouraged to exercise to exhaustion because this would be counterproductive. Muscle strength may be significantly improved by selected strengthening exercises under the supervision of a physical therapist. Swimming is an excellent athletic skill to learn early on because it provides full body exercise in an essentially weightless situation with which the weaker child can more easily cope.

Q: Are any types of alternative medical treatments effective in the treatment of muscular dystrophy?

A: Many have been tried, including acupuncture, herbal remedies, biomagnetic therapy, bodywork techniques, nutritional supplements, and the like. Unfortunately, none have proved beneficial.

Q: Can girls ever get a muscle disease that mimics DMD?

A: A female can express a Duchenne-like disease if she is a *manifesting carrier,* meaning that she has enough loss of muscle to exhibit weakness. Rarely, a female may have an abnormal X chromosome that causes what appears to be a disease like DMD. More frequently, a rapidly progressive autosomal recessive muscular dystrophy caused by a loss of one of the dystrophin-associated glycoproteins (molecules that function with dystrophin at the muscle membrane) may lead to a severe muscular dystrophy of childhood that can affect girls as well as boys.

Q: Can a DNA analysis of the blood always clinch the diagnosis of DMD?

A: Approximately two thirds of all cases of DMD can be diagnosed by DNA analysis. The remainder have an abnormality in their genes that requires a muscle biopsy for diagnosis.

Q: How can I tell whether my son has DMD or Becker muscular dystrophy (BMD)?

A: Becker muscular dystrophy usually is later in onset and less severe than DMD. Some doctors use the criterion of ability to walk unaided at age 16 years as a distinguishing sign of BMD. A more definitive test is the analysis of the protein dystrophin on a muscle biopsy—absent in DMD, diminished and/or aberrant in BMD. Some boys cannot be classified easily; they are called "Duchenne outliers" or "severe Beckers."

An important point about BMD is that severe cardiac involvement may accompany mild skeletal muscle weakness. Life expectancy in DMD is at best limited to the thirties; some men with BMD live well into adulthood and father children. These individuals should be aware that the X-linked nature of the condition puts all their daughters at 100 percent risk of being carriers but spares all sons from inheriting the disease.

3

THE DIAGNOSIS OF MUSCULAR DYSTROPHY

The very early diagnosis of muscular dystrophy frequently is missed. When there is no family history of the disease to alert the doctor to its possibility, children often are simply regarded as slow and clumsy. In one study a significant number of children examined for the first time were diagnosed as having a variety of foot problems, such as flat feet. Minimal signs of evolving weakness often are overlooked. These include flat feet (the result of heel cord tightness), weak shoulder extension, hesitance when ascending stairs, a slight pelvic shift to the side when arising from a seated position on the floor, a tendency to get up "butt first," acceleration during the final stage of sitting down (the so-called "plop-sit"), poor standing jump, and a tendency to waddle when running.

Later evidence of the disease is more apparent. Children waddle when they walk and fall frequently.

They have difficulty ascending stairs and "slip through" at the shoulders when lifted with support in their armpits. They now clearly climb up their bodies when rising from the floor. This is called a positive Gowers' (tripod) sign (Figure 3-1). Other physical findings are an increase in spinal lumbar lordosis (swayback), progressive equinus (drop foot) with toe-walking, calf hypertrophy (enlargement) (Figure 3-2), weak neck extension (straightening), and finally depression of all deep tendon reflexes (contraction of a muscle following "tapping" of a tendon).

FIGURE 3–1   The positive Gowers' tripod sign.

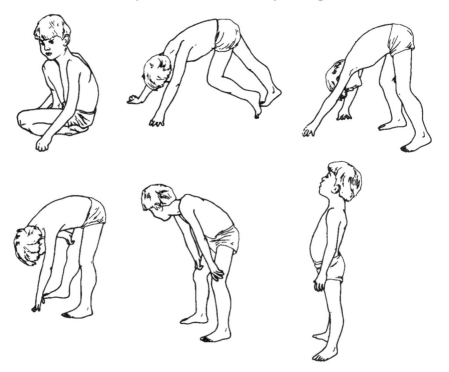

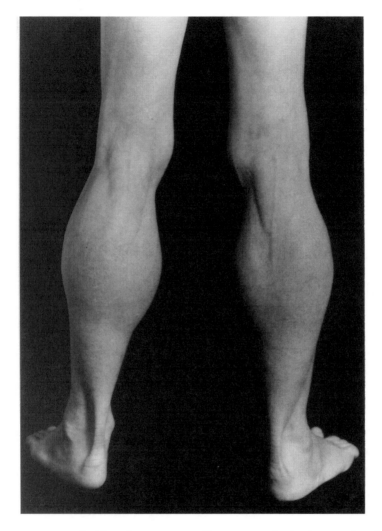

FIGURE 3–2   Calf enlargement (hypertrophy). An early sign of muscular dystrophy.

The diagnosis of muscle disease is made on the basis of a clinical history, physical examination, genetic evaluation, and laboratory studies that include muscle enzymes, electromyography, and muscle biopsy.

HISTORY

Your doctor will take a detailed history. Generally speaking, the symptoms of neuromuscular disease are those of weakness. How long has the weakness been present? What exacerbates or relieves it? Is it constant or intermittent? Progressive or diminishing? Are there associated symptoms such as pain?

Particularly important in the history is the timing of "motor milestones" (significant points in motor development—sitting, standing, walking, and the like), which often are delayed in the child with a neuromuscular condition. For example, 50 percent of children with Duchenne muscular dystrophy fail to walk until 18 months of age. Other questions are: Was the child hypotonic (floppy) during infancy? Are there complaints of cramps and stiffness? Pregnancy and birth usually are normal except that some mothers report diminished fetal movements. Has there been any exposure to extrinsic causes of muscle weakness, such as organic or inorganic toxins, trauma, drugs, or infections? Has the child's motor, language, and adaptive social behavior been normal? And, most important, because many neuromuscular diseases are hereditary, is there a family history of a similar disease?

PHYSICAL EXAMINATION

Children may be evaluated during play, when coordination and balance can be noted. The enlarged muscle with "pseudohypertrophy" in Duchenne dystrophy is rubbery and firm, in contrast to the flabby feeling of an atrophied (wasted) muscle or the firm resilience of a normal one.

Infants are examined for head drop and evaluated for hypotonia ("floppiness"). The range of motion of all major joints is tested for contracture. Muscles may be percussed (tapped) to see if they respond with spasm or if they show a condition called *myoedema* (muscle swelling), which is found in hypothyroidism. Quantitative strength assessment is made of the major postural muscle groups, those of the shoulders, hips, knees, and ankles. The spine is inspected for scoliosis (curvature). This sometimes is obvious, with one hip and shoulder higher than the other. The tongue (a muscle not covered by skin) is observed for atrophy (wasting) and fasciculations (twitching), which would indicate a disease of nerve rather than muscle.

In general, *myopathies*—diseases of muscles— show proximal (shoulder and hip) weakness, whereas *neuropathies*—diseases of nerves—begin distally (away from the trunk). As a rule, weakness exceeds atrophy (wasting) in myopathies such as muscular dystrophies, whereas atrophy exceeds weakness in neuropathic disease, such as hereditary neuropathy.

Testing a child's functional abilities in performing a standard set of tasks provides an excellent evaluation of his state of motor well-being. The method used is recorded, as is the time taken to perform each task. Activities most usefully assessed—because they most frequently show abnormalities—are (1) rising from a seated position on the floor, (2) stepping onto an elevation, (3) rising from a chair, (4) hopping on the toes, (5) walking on the heels, and (6) raising the arms overhead. Functional status can be rated on a 10-step scale. This may help to direct subsequent treatment (Table 3-1).

TABLE 3-1. Assessment

The patient can be rated on a functional 10-step scale:

(a) Stage 1: Walks and climbs stairs without assistance (it takes 15 times as much energy to ascend a flight of ordinary stairs as it does to walk a level distance equal to the vertical height of the stairs)

(b) Stage 2: Walks and climbs stairs easily with aid of railing

(c) Stage 3: Walks and climbs stairs slowly with aid of railing

(d) Stage 4: Walks but cannot climb stairs

(e) Stage 5: Walks unassisted but cannot climb stairs or get out of chair

(f) Stage 6: Walks only with assistance or with braces

(g) Stage 7: In wheelchair, sits erect and can roll chair and perform bed and wheelchair activities of daily living

(h) Stage 8: In wheelchair, sits erect but is unable to perform bed and chair activities without assistance

(i) Stage 9: In wheelchair, sits erect only with support and is able to do only minimal activities of daily living

(j) Stage 10: In bed, cannot perform activities of daily living without assistance

---

The kinetic sequence of the scale provides a treatment format for the physical therapy program.

(a) In Stages 1 to 3, the patient is ambulating independently. Passive stretch of early lower extremity contractures may be necessary by Stage 3. Functional activities of daily living and ambulation are sufficient active exercise for Stages 1–3.

(b) Between Stages 5 and 6, lower extremity surgery is indicated because contractures lead to increased difficulty with antigravity activities. When contracture is minimal or absent, orthotic modifications or bracing alone may be sufficient to augment weakened knee extension and keep the patient ambulating. With fair quadriceps strength, the knee flexion moment can be decreased by an anteriorly placed cushioned (SACH type) heel or converted to an extension moment with an equinus (floor reaction) AFO.

(c) Ambulant patients in Stages 5 and 6 should not avoid activity or use a wheelchair except when absolutely necessary and then for only brief periods of time.

(d) Stage 7 should not be skipped because the patient is thus immediately condemned to Stage 10.

(e) When Stage 7 is reached, routine conditioning exercises are prescribed to retard disuse atrophy and maintain independence in wheelchair activities. Prophylactic treatment of scoliosis also is initiated at this time, as is a full program of respiratory therapy.

(f) Obesity usually is a problem after Stage 6.

(g) The closer a patient is to Stage 10, the more assistive devices he or she requires.

LABORATORY TESTS

The medical history and physical examination are augmented by certain laboratory tests. Most important of these is the blood test for CK. Creatine phosphokinase provides the most sensitive chemical index for the diagnosis of muscular dystrophy. However, it also is elevated after exercise and is higher in younger individuals, African Americans, and males. Creatine phosphokinase may rise after an intramuscular injection, a heart attack, an injury to muscle, a convulsion, a variety of inflammatory diseases, sleep deprivation, acute psychosis, and so forth. Therefore, tests for other chemicals or metabolites may be indicated to evaluate a child for a specific neuromuscular condition.

A variety of imaging techniques may assist the doctor in making the diagnosis. Ultrasound is a useful and practical tool for screening muscle for pathologic change. Computerized tomography (CT) and magnetic resonance imaging (MRI) are both valuable in the detection of structural alteration of muscle, particularly in deep muscles that are inaccessible to physical examination.

ELECTROPHYSIOLOGIC EXAMINATION

Electrophysiologic examination includes the measurement of the conduction velocity of nerve (NCV, the rate at which a nerve transmits an electrical impulse), which is altered in certain diseases of nerves. Electromyography (EMG) is a technique in which the electrical pattern is observed on an oscilloscope, amplified, listened to, and recorded as a tracing (the readout is similar to an electrocardiogram). The EMG is a valuable tool that is used to visualize the electrical activity in muscle and to determine whether it is normal or abnormal and, if it is abnormal, whether it shows the characteristics of a neuropathic or myopathic process.

MUSCLE BIOPSY

A muscle biopsy can be taken either with a large bore needle or through a small incision and is accomplished easily without serious effect on the child. It provides the clinician with a specimen that can be stained for various constituents and analyzed chemically or by a standard microscope, fluorescent techniques, or electron microscopy. Specific conditions show characteristic findings on biopsy. Nerve can be similarly examined.

GENETICS

Many neuromuscular disorders are hereditary and most are caused by the mutation of a single gene (monogenic). Since the discovery of the location of the gene for Duchenne muscular dystrophy by Kunkel and his colleagues in 1985, more than 60 other mutations that cause neuromuscular diseases have been detected, as well as many more gene deletions and "point mutations" (spot changes) in the genes of the mitochondria (energy-producing components) present in all cells. Therefore, a pedigree chart with a detailed family history is essential for proper diagnosis.

Having established a diagnosis, we now consider the management of childhood muscular dystrophy. For convenience we do this by stages—first early childhood, next prepuberty, then adolescence, and finally late-late problems.

4

Early Childhood (Ages 5 to 9 Years)

Early childhood is a time during which the child with muscular dystrophy begins to experience difficulty with running, stair-walking, and other motor skills. This is particularly true during periods of accelerating growth, when bones are growing rapidly and muscle development is not keeping up. The "scale effect" describes this phenomenon. A small increment in the length of an extremity leads to an increase in surface area that is the square of the increase in length. However, the volume of the extremity increases by the cube of the increase in length. Therefore, you can see that a small increase in length may lead to a disproportionate increase in volume (Figure 4-1). This places a greater demand on muscle that is weakened by disease.

At the same time it sometimes seems as if the child actually is becoming stronger. This occurs during those times when a child's natural processes of

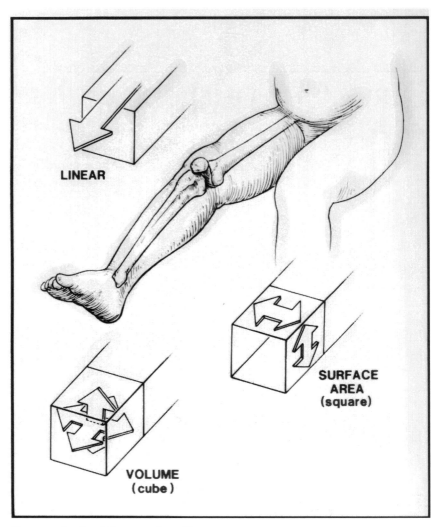

LINEAR

SURFACE
AREA
(square)

VOLUME
(cube)

FIGURE 4–1   The scale effect.

motor development outstrip the slow progress of the disease. Every 6-year-old has better motor skills than he had when he was 5. This is true of children with and without neuromuscular disease. Therefore, sometimes it seems as if the disease is arrested just because the child appears to be more coordinated.

The goals of physical therapy during this early stage are to enhance and protect muscular function for as long as possible. The physical therapy program addresses both *concentric* movements, which involve muscle *shortening* during movement, and *eccentric* movements, which involve muscle *lengthening* during movement.

Parents are the best advocates for their children, and they must find the balance between concentric activities such as bicycling and swimming and eccentric activities like running. Exercises are not formalized. Rather, they are introduced into the child's play activities. Swimming should be taught very early. It is an important skill to have and provides excellent non-stressful exercise. Heel cords and hips should be stretched on a daily basis when they begin to tighten. The use of night splints to inhibit heel cord contracture is controversial. If prescribed, their use must be initiated early and they should be worn every night. Bending the knees relaxes the heel cords. Therefore, to be most effective, night splints should reach from above the knees to the toes.

In selected cases a *tone-balancing brace* can stabilize the ankle, stretch the heel cord during walking, and inhibit the evolution of severe heel cord contracture, which challenges balance and prohibits standing. This short, light appliance easily fits into a standard soft shoe, can be covered by an ordinary sock, and is well tolerated (Figure 4-2).

Some physicians advocate extensive surgery to relieve incipient contractures of muscle, fascia, and tendons in the legs at approximately 5 years of age. This purportedly avoids the necessity for physical therapy, giving the patient a better quality of life.

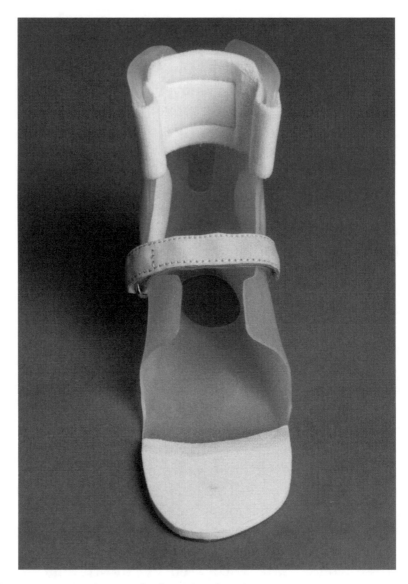

FIGURE 4–2   A tone-balancing brace.

However, the benefits of this radical surgery are questionable and physicians are reluctant to perform such operations on children who as yet have little difficulty walking.

Medications known as *corticosteroids* have been found to slow muscle degeneration in some cases of Duchenne muscular dystrophy. These drugs are given by mouth on a daily or alternating day schedule. Corticosteroids are potent antiinflammatory agents that have serious side effects, including weight gain; osteoporosis, which may lead to vertebral fracture; skin problems, including thinning of the skin and acne; cataracts; high blood pressure; susceptibility to infection; retention of salt and loss of potassium; redistribution of body fat; round puffy facial appearance; growth retardation; depression of immune response; an increase in blood sugar, which may lead to diabetes; and psychological problems, including emotional overstimulation. Research is being conducted on new corticosteroid drugs that may be as effective as those currently available but have fewer side effects.

Before a child is given a corticosteroid, it should be determined that he is not already an overeater and that he can handle reasonable dietary management. He should not be overactive or emotionally labile because the medication may make this worse.

Corticosteroids slow down muscle degradation but they do not cure the basic pathology. Many patients receiving corticosteroids eventually require surgery and/or bracing. The medication usually is not started earlier than the age of 5 years; the growth rate of younger children is greater, so their growth may be more impaired by corticosteroids; and children should have been through their childhood contagious infections and have completed their program of routine immunizations before beginning medication. All other things being equal, the use of carefully monitored corticosteroids in Duchenne muscular dystrophy is a viable option because it seems to prolong muscle strength and increase respiratory function.

Diet should be carefully monitored in the child with a neuromuscular disease. Proper nutrition is essential and obesity must be avoided. In particular, Duchenne muscular dystrophy is a rather fragile condition and excess weight may tax weakened muscles to the point that standing and ambulation may be inhibited.

PSYCHOLOGICAL ADJUSTMENT

The Patient

The adjustment of a child with muscular dystrophy may be affected by several factors, including:

(1) The requirement for parental separation at any time during the disease. Young children separated from parents for long periods of time show adverse reactions characterized by a stage of protest, followed by a stage of detachment or denial.

(2) Restriction, including sensory impairment and isolation. When the normal activities of expression through play are restricted, a child may withdraw into excessive fantasy as a means of coping.

(3) Lack of consistency and dependency.

(4) Medication. The prolonged, regular use of drugs may be regarded as an imposition by authority figures.

(5) Concerns over being defective; hence the fear of becoming an inadequate person.

(6) Absence from school.

(7) Threat of death. It usually is not until age 9 or 10 years that any child fully understands death as being both inevitable and irrevocable.

The Family

The following factors influence a family's response to the severe stress on the family unit coping with the diagnosis and treatment of a chronic illness in one of its members.

(1) The severity of the illness, including both the prognosis and the availability of an effective treatment.

(2) Whether the disease is congenital.

(3) The onset of the disease and the age at which the diagnosis is made.

(4) The presence of a preexisting emotional disturbance within the family.

(5) The nature and effects of the illness itself.

(6) The effects of a program of home management and restrictions on family life.

(7) The presence or absence of affected siblings.

(8) The stress of repeated hospitalizations.

(9) The cost of the illness if privately treated.

Parents

Specific emotional responses seen in parents include denial, anxiety, feelings of guilt, depression, resentment (and rejection), and reactions of shame, embarrassment, or sheer exhaustion.

Many parents evolve through the various stages of mourning after learning the diagnosis. This includes a period of disbelief and denial, succeeded by one of anger and rage, followed by bargaining and, finally, acceptance and adjustment. There are a number of critical psychosocial incidents in DMD. These include diagnosis, inability of the patient to cope, bracing, wheelchair confinement, and so forth, and parents may reinitiate the mourning process at each of these events.

Siblings

Sibling reactions are more or less characterized by similar emotional states. Normal siblings often feel responsible for their diseased sibling and/or guilty over their own normality. Indeed, muscular dystrophy may largely form the basis for a family's way of life. Because of the demands of the illness, siblings become handicapped in the struggle for parental affection and attention.

A sibship is unique in that it may span six or more decades. Siblings identify closely with each other. They may feel responsible for each other's well-being. The healthy child must be aided in developing his own identity and in understanding the differences and similarities between himself and his disabled sibling. Systematic and routine inquiry should be made into the effect the illness may be having on normal siblings. Specific information should be sought regarding peer relationships, academic progress, sleep, mood, and the like. What the sibling needs is empathy, not sympathy. Whereas the child with muscular dystrophy should know that "everybody's different, nobody's perfect" the sibling who is shouting "Hey, I'm here too!" requires ongoing concern and attention even though his anxiety and occasional anger may be borne silently. Literature and psychosocial support in these matters are available through MDA.

School

A close liaison should be maintained between parents and doctor and/or clinic with the child's school. Children spend more than half of their waking hours in a classroom. School is essential not only for academic growth but also for emotional and social development. Children evaluate themselves in large part in the school setting. Here they judge their academic achievements, interact with peers, and are evaluated through the eyes of their teachers.

If the message the child receives in school is one of acceptance and the atmosphere in the classroom encourages striving for excellence, the school—through the teacher—may play a major role in helping establish a child's positive outlook toward his life.

Teachers should be informed about the details of a child's signs and symptoms, his rate of progression, and the problems they may pose in the school setting.

Ultimately, some adaptations at school may be necessary. These may include such items as a raised toilet seat, a special desktop, and a laptop computer. For many students with neuromuscular diseases, having a one-on-one aide in the classroom provides the best solution. Each pupil should have an individualized education plan that considers his or her special needs. Federal and state laws require schools to provide the modifications that are needed for disabled students to attend school.

Teachers should know that a child's developing weakness may make it difficult for him to take notes quickly or over a long period of time. He may be slow in preparing for class and getting his materials in order. Using a computer may speed up things. A supportive teacher-student relationship may relieve a child's anxiety and allow discussion of his feelings in a nonthreatening environment.

Teachers should also understand that although some children with DMD suffer cognitive difficulty, most are of average intelligence and some are even of above-average intelligence. When cognitive problems exist, they usually are in the area of verbal learning. It is important to recognize that even if the child with DMD has a cognitive problem, it will be nonprogressive in nature.

Except in extreme conditions the child should be mainstreamed in his local school. This is important because school provides a rich opportunity for social interaction with his peers and adults other than members of his own family. In the classroom situation the child should, as far as possible, be treated as an equal with his fellow students. As with all children, praise for accomplishments and emphasis on abilities is desirable. Discipline should be consistent. Every child should believe he is important and also should know that rules and behavioral limits are to be respected.

QUESTIONS

Q: Do the arms also weaken in Duchenne muscular dystrophy?

A: Weakness of the muscles of the shoulder is present early in the disease. In fact, the muscles that extend (draw back) the shoulders are among the first to be affected. However, weakness in the arms does not advance as rapidly as weakness in the legs because the arms are not under as much stress as the legs because of their involvement in maintaining posture. Weakness in the arms causes no real problems in the early stages of DMD.

Q: Is there any pain associated with Duchenne muscular dystrophy?

A: Other than occasional mild cramping in the calves early in the disease, little or no pain is associated with DMD. In fact, there is no effect on sensation in general.

Q: How much should the child know about his disease?

A: Children are able to cope better in an environment that facilitates truthful communication. The child should know as much about his disease and treatment as possible. His questions should be answered truthfully in a way that is commensurate with his ability to understand. Information should be shared with all family members and caregivers. This includes close friends and teachers. Openness with the child and all who are involved with his care is of vital importance.

Q: How can a teacher respond to classmates' questions concerning the child's disease?

A: The sincere and sensitive teacher who encourages a child to feel comfortable about asking questions and expressing feelings will be able to handle this through an open discussion in the classroom. When classmates understand the child's disability and needs, they are less likely to tease and more liable to assist the child and become his advocates.

Q: Can a child with muscular dystrophy participate in physical education?

A: Physical education is an important aspect of any child's school experience. For social as well as physical reasons, the child should be encouraged and allowed to participate. This may be accomplished by providing lighter weight equipment, assistance from a helper, or even allowing the child to be the scorekeeper or manager during team sports.

Q: Does DMD affect the mind?

A: The average IQ for children with DMD is within normal range and does not decline with time. People with DMD often attend college and subsequently find work. At the same time, the IQ of about 10 percent of all patients falls approximately 10 percent below normal, and deficits in expressive language and verbal comprehension often present as dyslexia. The mental impairment in DMD is unrelated to the physical problems of the disease and is not progressive.

Q: What about play? What toys are appropriate for the child with DMD?

A: Playing is an important learning experience. Group play should be encouraged because it is a vital part of social development. A full range of adaptive sports equipment for children with disabilities is available. Creative play is especially important and you can introduce your child to all kinds of physically undemanding activities such as reading, writing, crafts, art, music, gardening, photography, collecting, and computer games, which he can continue to enjoy throughout his life.

Q: What is the best philosophy for raising a child with a disability?

A: Live in the here and now and make each day count. Don't forget that your child is a child first and a child with a disability second. You have to encourage independence and learn to let go. This involves some risk-taking but it is a wise investment in your child's sense of self-worth. Be open and honest and let the child know each day that you love him and are there to care for him as you would for any child of yours, disabled or not.

Q: How can I help my son with DMD feel less disabled and more normal?

A: By providing him with the opportunity to have normal experiences. These may include family outings, carefully planned travel and camping, suitable recreation, and the like. Don't get so involved with your son's medical requirements that you ignore the important fact that children need to have fun, and families need to share.

5

PREPUBERTY (AGES 9 TO 12 YEARS)

The muscles that form first in the embryo—the spinal musculature and muscles of the shoulders and hips— are initially and most severely involved in DMD (Figure 5-1). Most large muscles of the body require a loss of at least 30 percent to 40 percent of their structure before clinical weakness is evident. This fact accounts for the apparent normal functioning of children with DMD during the first years of life. On average it takes a child 4.8 years to lose approximately half of his or her muscle strength. The apparent improvement in some children from 5 to 7 years of age can be explained by the processes of normal development outstripping progression of the disease during this period; the mechanical efficiency of the skeleton probably doubles as the body normally matures.

A greater proportion of muscle is required as the limbs grow. This explains why a child with a condition that limits his ultimate mass initially may be ambula-

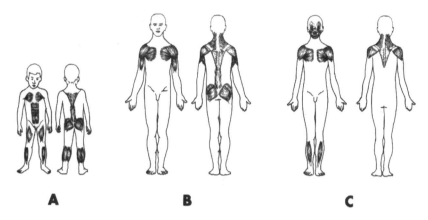

A   **B**   **C**

FIGURE 5–1   Early distribution of muscle weakness in the three major forms of muscular dystrophy. (**A**) Duchenne dystrophy (**B**) Limb-girdle dystrophy (**C**) Facioscapulohumeral dystrophy.

tory but eventually loses the ability to walk as he develops. Below the age of 7.5 years there is little or no functional change over a single year in 75 percent of boys with DMD. Beyond age 7.5 years 75 percent show significant functional change every year.

At approximately age 7.5 years a child begins to realize that he is different from other children because of increasing difficulty with motor tasks. Beginning at age 9 years the average child with DMD will begin to have trouble ascending stairs, rising from the seated position, and walking; these changes tend to occur in roughly that sequence at yearly intervals. There is a close congruence with affected brothers regarding the ability to perform these tasks.

Three processes contribute to the deformities of muscular dystrophy: muscle weakness, muscle imbalance, and specific muscle contractures that develop as the result of compensatory postural habits in response to gravity. Contracture often is asymmetric and less in the dominant limb. At this stage it is desirable to maintain physical function through an aggressive program of physical therapy that includes supervised appropriate exercise such as gait training and transfer techniques as well as contracture stretching, particularly of hip flexors, knees, and heel cords (Table 5-1). Proper physical therapy should preserve the balance necessary for maintenance of upright posture. The child with muscle disease must be kept physically active for as long as possible. Standing and walking are the best functional therapy for accomplishing this. A minimum of 2 to 3 hours a day of such activity is encouraged. If the child is rested after a full night's sleep, he is not being overexercised.

TABLE 5–1.	Exercises for Stretching Key Musculature	
Muscles	*Active*	*Passive*
Hip flexors	Lying face up at edge of table, hold opposite knee and hip bent up, drop leg over edge and allow weight of leg to stretch back	Child lying face down— knees straight. While holding hip from behind, elevate knee from the table
Tensor fascia (iliotibial band)	Stand with one side toward wall and feet about 8–12 inches from the wall. Keep knees straight and lean the near hip toward the wall	Child lying face down—thigh bent back and to the side. Holding hip firmly from behind, bring thigh toward the body to maximum stretch position
Hamstrings	Toe-touching in standing or seated position with the knees straight	Child lying face up, hip bent up, knee straight, elevate leg to maximum stretch position

TABLE 5–1. *(continued)*

Muscles	Active	Passive
Heel cords	Stand arm's length from a wall. Supporting body with hands on wall and keeping hands on wall and keeping knees straight and *heels on the floor* attempt to lean chest to wall, thus bending ankles up	Child lying face up with knees straight. Cup heel in palm, inverting (twisting in) foot to lock joints of the foot and supporting sole to avoid bending the middle of the foot. Bend ankle up to position of maxmimal stretch

The child with DMD uses certain postural adaptations to enable his body to remain upright. These involve modulating his center of gravity (CG) within its base of support. To do this, he must hyperextend (bend back) his hips and extend (straighten) his knees. Knee stability is assisted by toe-walking, and increasing lumbar lordosis (swayback) helps to balance the torso over the pelvis.

Because muscles work in pairs, as the hip extensors weaken, the hip flexors contract; and when the muscles that dorsiflex (bring up) the ankle weaken, the heel cords contract. With progressive weakness and contracture, standing and walking become increasingly laborsome. Functional loss increases and the center of gravity can no longer be modulated through compensatory posture. A vicious cycle in which fibrotic muscle shortening leading to contracture and deformity with unequal weakness results in increased atrophy and imbalance requiring further compensatory posturing, leading to increased fibrotic muscle shortening, and so forth is set in motion (Figure 5-2).

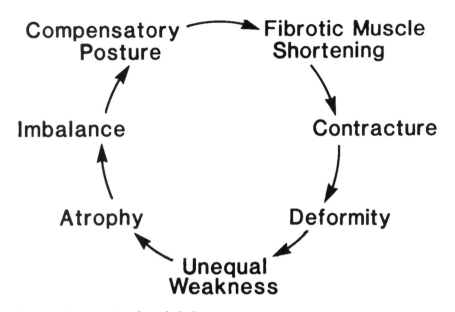

FIGURE 5–2 Cycle of deformity.

Muscles that control posture through a dynamic reflex mechanism degenerate into static supportive structures that are vulnerable to imposed stress and subsequently waste and contract. The child has increased difficulty managing those momentary imbalances that occur during ambulation. Generalized weakness makes it increasingly difficult to attain alignment and stability when an attempt is made to balance the trunk over unstable lower extremities. Sufficient strength is lacking to execute those postural adjustments necessary to compensate for weakening and contracture (Figure 5-3).

Small nonmuscular changes assume significance at this time. A slight weight gain or a period of several days of bedrest (when strength is lost at 3 percent to 5 percent a day) may increase weakness enough to impair ambulation. Duchenne muscular dystrophy is a disease that is sensitive to minor changes in a child's physical state, and the transition from moderately to severely impaired ambulation may be abrupt. Because of individual differences in weakness, contracture, weight, and motivation, age alone is a poor index of disease progression. The more disabled the child, the more determinants of gait are lost, the more energy is required for ambulation, and the less efficient is the gait.

FIGURE 5–3   The development of functional loss as the result of weakening and contracture.

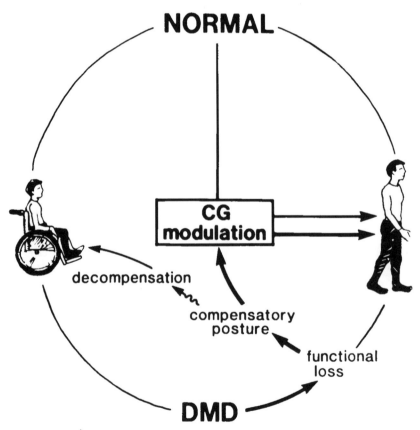

Before the child stops walking entirely, long leg braces (occasionally short leg braces if the knees are strong enough) may be beneficial in maintaining the upright posture and permitting continued walking. Surgery may be necessary to fit these braces. The aim of this surgery is to release ambulation-limiting contractures—usually of the hips, the knees, and the heel cords (Figure 5-4)—sufficiently to maintain adequate standing and walking equilibrium. Surgery must permit early postoperative mobilization. Even brief restraint may lead to rapid loss of strength; it is difficult, if not impossible, to regain the ability to stand and walk once the child uses a wheelchair.

SURGERY

Operative release of contractures can be performed with a fine instrument called a *tenotome* through a small puncture wound in the skin. Blood loss is minimal and sutures are unnecessary. The procedure takes only a few minutes. Lightweight long leg plaster casts are applied so that the child can stand and walk

FIGURE 5–4   Sites of contracture release: (1) hip flexors, (2) and (3) tensor fascia, and (4) heel cord.

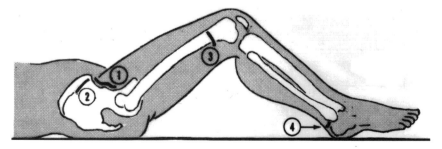

immediately after the operation. If the knees are strong enough, a short plaster cast may be used. Patients walk in these casts for 3 weeks, at which time braces are fitted. Sometimes braces can be measured and fabricated before surgery. They are then worn instead of plaster casts.

These surgical procedures usually are indicated between 9 and 12 years of age (occasionally earlier or later) and may be performed on an outpatient basis. No hospitalization is required. A light general anesthetic is required. It is important that the anesthesiologist be experienced in the management of the child with a muscle disease who may be a poor anesthetic risk. Such children sometimes have inadequate pulmonary reserve and run the risk of malignant hyperthermia, a condition in which temperature rapidly elevates to a dangerous level. A medication called *dantrolene* may be given prophylactically to prevent malignant hyperthermia. Should hyperthermia occur during surgery, intravenous dantrolene will abort an attack.

Another operation that sometimes is performed to prevent deformity of the ankle is to *transect* or transfer the tendon of the posterior tibia, a muscle that twists the ankle and foot in, making it difficult for the child to walk. The tendon is either simply cut or transferred to the outer aspect of the top of the foot, where it will now work to pull the foot up and out rather than down and in.

ORTHOSES

All orthoses (braces) are made of vacuum-molded plastic. These appliances are considerably lighter but as sturdy as their steel or aluminum counterparts.

The plastic brace incorporates a molded footplate that easily fits into any footwear. This includes tennis shoes or running shoes, which are the most desirable footwear for the child with DMD because of their lightness and scored rubber soles, which grip the floor. Ankle mobility in the brace may be regulated by varying the width of the posterior strut connecting the calf portion to the footplate. Because the appliance is form-fitted from plastic, it is less bulky than a standard metal brace, more comfortable, and cosmetically acceptable. It may be worn under an ordinary stocking and does not require special clothing adaptations. Velcro fittings are used for closure, or a singular tubular construction may be prescribed that uses even thinner plastic because the tubular form is more resistant to superimposed stress than the open model (Figure 5-5). Knee hinges are used so that the knees can bend for sitting. All materials used in these orthoses are nontoxic, radiolucent (X-ray transparent), unaffected by oils or ultraviolet light, and completely waterproof. The appliances can be washed and dried with ease.

Because of their lightness, ease of application and removal, cosmetic acceptability, and other advantages, there is strong patient compliance and parental satisfaction with these braces.

Physical therapy after surgery consists mostly of walking. The braces are worn at night for 6 weeks, after which time they may be removed during sleep.

Patients who continue to walk in braces maintain better alignment of weight-bearing joints and suffer less wasting of bone and disuse of muscle than those who are not ambulatory. Through surgery and bracing, the vicious cycle of weakness-imbalance-contrac-

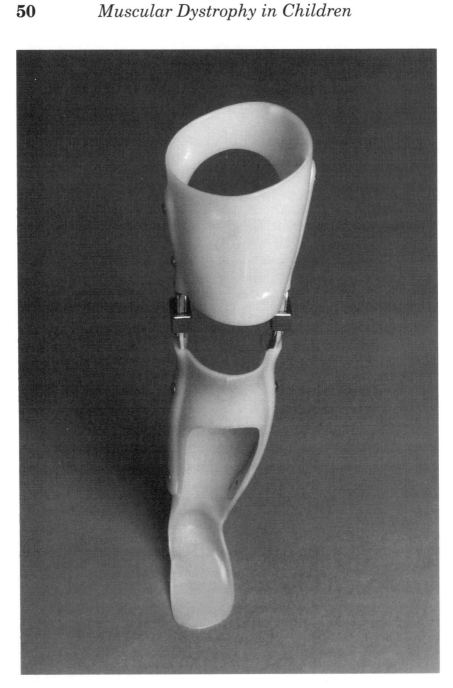

FIGURE 5–5   A plastic molded knee-ankle-foot brace.

ture-deformity in muscular dystrophy can be broken, delaying progression of disability.

More than half of a child's total muscle mass is lost by the end of independent ambulation, when he sometimes is too weak to stand alone. However, he often is able to walk again after correction of contractures and bracing because other factors also are influential in preventing ambulation. These causes include obesity, emotional problems, and, most of all, intermittent wheelchair immobilization imposed for the convenience of others. After surgery and bracing, a patient usually can handle his toilet needs with minimal help and facilitate transfer when his braces are locked at the knees and his legs are used as a long lever to tilt him to the standing position. The additional period of independent ambulation and therapeutic standing attained through these procedures is usually 2 to 4 years beyond the time a child would normally require a wheelchair.

As is apparent, the rule here is, "less is more"—the object is to perform minimal surgery and get the patient up and walking immediately after his operation. Downtime should be kept to a minimum, and most children can return to school a few days after their operation.

FRACTURES

There is no disorder of mineral metabolism in Duchenne muscular dystrophy. The child's bones are normal in structure, but because of inactivity they become thin and break easily. It is said that muscular dystrophy is a disease in which the soft tissues get hard and the hard tissues get soft. A fall may cause a fracture, usually in a long bone such as those of the arms or legs. The most severe fractures are seen in wheelchair-using patients who fall from the chair rather than in patients who are still walking. There usually is minimal displacement of bone fragments and often less pain than with a fracture in a normal child because there is little muscle spasm. All fractures heal without complication and within the expected time interval. The danger of restrictive procedures in children with DMD must be recognized, and their fractures should be treated with minimal splintage. Light plaster casts should be used, and the patient should be allowed to stand and walk as soon as possible. The key to success is "less is more." Use light support and maintain ambulation.

OCCUPATIONAL THERAPY

Occupational therapy (OT) is important at this stage to evaluate the home environment for possible adaptations. These may include an elevated toilet seat, bathtub rails, or adaptive eating equipment. The Muscular Dystrophy Association publishes literature on simple measures that may be employed at home to facilitate tasks of daily living. Some adaptations may be necessary at school, and the child may find it necessary to use a wheelchair part-time while at school. As muscles weaken, stairs, long distances, and doors becomes obstacles. The student may have to use an elevator to get from class to class. Doorways must be wide enough for a wheelchair if it is used, and toileting privacy should be provided. Because the child with DMD is experiencing a decrease in his ability to control physical activities, it is important for him to continue to feel in control by allowing him choices.

Architectural barriers both at home and in the community often pose a problem. Anticipating difficulty with stairs, it is prudent to plan, when possible, to have the child's bedroom, bathroom, and play needs available on the first floor. A single-level (ranch-style) home is best. If there are no bathing facilities on the first floor in a two-level home, a chair lift can be arranged to transport the child to the second floor.

PSYCHOSOCIAL NEEDS

Children with DMD tend to be emotionally dependent and some cannot tolerate frustration. They may slip toward social and emotional withdrawal and exhibit emotional seesawing and impulsive responses. Parents must be aware of the emotional crisis that occurs when a child senses he is different from other children, particularly when this difference manifests as an inability to keep up—much less compete—physically. In general, parents can only understand what they are emotionally prepared for. In dealing with the psychological problems of both the patient and his normal siblings, it is important to learn to read between the lines, to "listen to the music" and not to the words, and to sense and deal with the child's feelings (anxiety, fear, guilt, frustration, and the like), whether directly or indirectly expressed.

Understanding and communication may be facilitated by family or individual psychotherapy. This need not be intense or prolonged. Often just a few sessions can clear the air and lead to significant insights and an increased ability to understand and deal with emotional problems in the home.

QUESTIONS

Q: What are the major psychological problems of adjustment facing parents of children with DMD?

A: Feelings of guilt may lead to penance and a life of servitude to the child and may contribute to a vicious cycle of guilt, anger, self-pity, and ultimate rejection, both of self and of the child. Demands on the mother's time and strength are severe. Neighbors are not always tactful, and strangers provoke self-consciousness and shame. Normal siblings often are neglected. A major part of a counselor's job is to help parents realize the prospects of the child with DMD and his home situation as well as his limitations, and to aid siblings who have to compete with a sick child for parental attention.

Q: What are some of the therapeutic implications of understanding the emotional needs of the patient with DMD and his family?

A: Parents should be encouraged to focus more of their attention and energy on each other and on the unaffected children in the family. It is desirable to have increased earlier involvement of fathers in the care of the child. Marital stability is of the utmost importance. This requires effort on the part of both parents as they consider and work on all aspects of the marital relationship. The amount of physical labor demanded of the parents (the mother in particular) should be alleviated. If at all possible, child care services must be made available. Parents are constantly reworking their coping tasks. They must realize that progressive integration of parental roles and gradual acceptance of necessary tasks facilitate adaptation to their new life-style. Adjustment does not occur overnight.

Q: What is the best way to deal with the emotional problems of a child with DMD?

A: Most people tend to talk too much. Learn how to listen well, how to "tune in" to a child's problems, and how to "read between the lines." A child's most common worries should be discussed. This includes concern over the trouble he might be causing others in the family. The judicious use of aids for daily living may increase a child's independence and go far toward alleviating such concerns. One of the most difficult things is to try not to be overprotective. Even though you have no ready solution for every difficulty, just indicating that you recognize the problem can go a long way toward solving it. Learn to use your intuition. When a child inquires about his disease, including its fatal aspect, he must be given answers that are realistic and hopeful, at a level commensurate with his understanding. It is important to recognize exactly what the child is asking and to respond to this specific request for information, not to one's own anxieties and fantasies. During the early course of the disease, the child should be asked what he has been told by his teachers, siblings, and peers. A frank discussion of his concerns should be initiated. The child has to be encouraged to unburden himself of fears and fantasies, and every caretaker must be a good listener.

Q: Are there any methods besides surgery and long-leg bracing to keep a patient upright and walking?

A: Sometimes neoprene knee sleeves reinforced with metal stays can stabilize the knees enough to prolong standing and walking for many months. Occasionally a light below-knee brace may help.

Q: Is any specific physical therapy or occupational therapy useful at this stage of the disease?

A: The occupational therapist continues to evaluate the home environment for safety and accessibility. The activities and exercises of the early phase should be continued. Other activities could include therapeutic horseback riding, basketball, soccer, playful wrestling on the floor with an adult, and the like. Such exercises develop the balance-maintaining compensatory movements that a child requires to continue walking.

The use of night splints to control heel cord contracture is controversial. To be effective, they should be used early and continuously. Children often resist wearing them. On balance, a good night's rest is more important than the use of splints.

Q: Are respiratory and cardiac evaluation and care necessary at this time?

A: Active children usually don't have serious respiratory problems. However, it is wise to obtain a respiratory evaluation as a baseline and to encourage the child in activities that use his lungs and increase their capacity. These include singing, playing a wind instrument (even a kazoo or harmonica), blowing up balloons, and so forth. The chest muscles, like those of the arms and legs, tend to tighten without regular use. This stiffening can limit respiration. That is why it is important for the child to perform deep breathing exercises. Inoculation against flu and pneumonia is strongly recommended. Upper respiratory tract infections should be zealously avoided (this requires avoiding exposure to sudden shifts of temperature or extreme cold, having proper humidification in the home, particularly in the bedroom where a child sleeps, and so on). If a respiratory tract infection occurs, it must be treated vigorously with an appropriate antibiotic.

The heart is a muscle and is affected by the disease process in a significant number of DMD patients. However, the cardiac problems of DMD patients are alleviated by their diminished muscle mass, which reduces the load on the circulation. Cardiac function should be checked regularly, starting from the age of 10 to 12 years, to identify the occasional child with an early cardiac problem. The majority of children have no clinical cardiac difficulty during this stage of the disease. As far as monitoring cardiac function, the diagnostic value of a standard electrocardiogram is limited. Special tests such as echocardiography provide more prognostic information.

6

ADOLESCENCE

Illness in adolescence is resented as a particularly painful cheating of someone who is about to experience all of the supposed freedoms and opportunities that go along with being an adult. Adolescence is a time of change for all children. The physical and emotional changes that the youngster is experiencing are challenging to him, his peers, and his family and teachers. When viewed in the broader perspective, knowing that these changes are a normal part of the transition from childhood to young adulthood, from dependence to independence, makes these difficulties tolerable and even welcome.

The child with muscular dystrophy is faced with a difficult situation. His evolving weakness frustrates his attempts at physical independence. As his friends prepare for the challenges of life, including having a family and making vocational choices, the adolescent with DMD faces a life that offers fewer options and perhaps a limited life expectancy.

Progressive weakness may limit the ability of the adolescent to handle his tasks of daily living and establish meaningful social relationships. He often must be cared for like a younger child. These problems may be addressed in a variety of ways. Having a friend assist with classwork, eating, and even toileting is one possibility. What is most important, however, is to allow the child to help decide how his problems will be managed at home and at school. Input from all caretakers is necessary, including that of medical personnel, but the final decision must have the child's approval.

During the period of early adolescence it is important that the youngster stand and walk as much as possible (at least 2 hours each day). Because children are seated in a classroom during the school day, and frequently moved in a wheelchair because this is more convenient, it is essential that the child be encouraged to stand and walk when at home. If the school will cooperate, the student may stand during recess and even for brief periods of time during the school day.

Adaptive equipment such as hydraulic or electric lifts and ramps, or other architectural modifications in the home, may be necessary at this time. Work simplification techniques are taught. A counter and hip-level "bar stool" with a back, arm rests, and a foot rung will make it easier for the child to sit and stand up with minimal assistance so that he will be less hesitant to socialize at home. With enough residual strength, some adolescents can even drive a car adapted for the disabled.

TABLE 6–1. Adaptive Aids and Assistive Devices

1. Easy-lift chair	Assists patient to standing position
2. Bathroom grab bars	For standing and transfer
3. Clothing adaptations	Utilizing easily manipulated Velcro fastenings, special zippers on trousers, large socks with elastic tops, oversized-buttoned shirt, etc., for easy manipulation and facilitation of independence and self-care
4. Foot boards	To diminish heel cord contracture
5. Over-bed cradles	To keep covers off the legs for comfort, enabling the patient to move freely in bed without fighting the weight of blankets
6. Reachers	For patients with arm weakness
7. Hydraulic or electric lifts	For use in transfer to and from chair, bed, bath, etc.
8. Inlay-depth shoe with deerskin uppers	For foot comfort and stability
9. Balanced forearm orthosis (ball-bearing feeders)	To assist eating and other fine motor skills in wheelchair-confined patient
10. Button hooks	Of value to patient with loss of fine finger movement
11. Wrist extension splint	For wrist stability
12. Extension-handle utensils	To eliminate the need for lifting the forearm in patient with arm weakness
13. Wheelchair cushion	Most frequently used are "eggcrate" foam, silicone gel, and solid seat foam insert
14. Alternating pressure mattress, waterbed, special foam mattress	To assist in alleviating body pressure during sleep
15. Nylon sheets and pajamas	Facilitate position changes in bed by decreasing friction of movement
16. Raised chairs or toilet seat	Requires less hip and knee extensor strength in rising

TABLE 6–1. *(Continued)*

17. Doorknob extensions	Increases lever arm of doorknob
18. Built-up handle eating utensils	To provide improved grasp
19. Wheelchair lap trays	To provide conveniently placed work surface
20. Transfer boards	For sliding transfer from wheelchair to car or bed

Realistic preparation for college and an anticipated vocation are important. In addition to maintaining range of motion, it is important to address equipment needs, including telephone aids to maintain social contact and special adaptive equipment (Table 6-1) to compensate for severe motor loss.

The child with DMD often can excel at intellectual pursuits. Computers are popular because they require skill, not strength. Computer studies should be encouraged. Office-type armrests are available to support arms and hands over the keyboard. Roller balls on the mouse facilitate access to computer functions.

USE OF A WHEELCHAIR

In late adolescence many children spend some time in a manual wheelchair, particularly when they are traveling outside the home. A lightweight manual wheelchair will be needed for transportation to school or family outings. The wheelchair should be used only to expedite transport over a distance, and standing and walking must continue to be encouraged.

A power wheelchair is necessary when a child lacks the strength to stand and walk independently and cannot move a manual wheelchair by himself. This is not the beginning of the end, just the beginning of a new period in life. One of the advantages of surgery and bracing is that they delay the need for a wheelchair. Another is that the patient wearing long leg braces can be managed more effectively when using a wheelchair. The braces balance and seat him in the chair. They inhibit heel cord contracture, and they can be used to stretch the knees. When locked, he or she can be tilted to the upright position or into a pivot-shift transfer. This simple transfer technique is taught by a physical therapist. It is much easier to move a patient from chair to bed or toilet this way than having to lift his or her body weight from the chair.

Loss of the ability to walk, making use of a wheelchair necessary, is a critical incident in the life of the child with muscular dystrophy, both physiologically and psychologically. Every effort should be devoted to making the wheelchair a passport to *more* activity rather than less.

Special wheelchair adaptations may increase comfort while providing spinal support. Wheelchair prescriptions should not be regarded casually. The wheelchair is an *orthosis* (brace) and should be treated as such. Its prescription and fabrication should be supervised by a seating specialist. Proper fit is vital. If the wheelchair is too wide, the child will lean to one side, facilitating the development of scoliosis; if it is too deep, a kyphotic (round back) posture is encouraged. Seating includes standardized modules and custom-contoured seating such as the Contour-U® or Silhouette® external spinal containment systems, which seat the patient squarely in the chair and support the back (Figure 6-1).

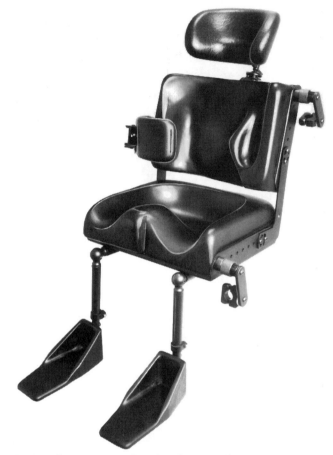

FIGURE 6–1   An external spinal containment system to attain proper posture while seated in a wheelchair.

Adequate trunk support can position the patient upright, enabling him to use a wheelchair more effectively. A firm seat and back and a wide chest and pelvic safety belt are provided. If weak neck extension is a problem, an extended back rest will be fitted to support the head. The wheelchair must be of proper size, with the narrowest seat width possible that gives full support.

It should be the correct height from the floor. It should incorporate wide front and rear tires for various terrains; handbrakes; angle adjustable, removable, elevating, swinging footrests with heel straps located so that there is no pressure behind the knees; upholstered removable desklike arms; and good brakes. The back support must not inhibit shoulder or elbow motion while it balances the trunk over the hips. A recliner back should be considered to allow for a change of position for part of the day to stretch out hip contractures. The tilt-in-space feature on manual and power wheelchairs permits an easy change of position to relieve low back and pelvic pressure without removing the child from the chair. This feature is especially helpful in school.

Additional wheelchair adaptations include balanced forearm orthoses. These are articulated forearm supports that enable weakened upper extremity muscles to operate *across* rather than *against* the field of gravity, facilitating the use of the hands for self-feeding, writing, and other useful tasks such as using a word processor or computer. They also include lapboards and over-bed tilt-top tables to provide a comfortably positioned work surface.

To avoid contractures, it is important that the hips, knees, and ankles be passively stretched every day. Tightness in the hamstring muscles (behind the knee) may lead to hip extensor contracture, which in turn causes pelvic rotation and sitting on the base of the spine. This posture requires contortion of the upper spine with forward head thrust for balance. Hamstring tightening is a major cause of pelvic displacement in the wheelchair user.

A combination wheelchair-commode eliminates the problem of difficult toilet transfers. The development of disabling contractures of the lower extremities may be delayed by using adjustable angle footrests or foot wedges that hold the ankles at neutral or in slight dorsiflexion (bent up) as well as extended (straightened) legrests to prevent flexion contracture of the knees.

Significant psychological and physiologic value is obtained from standing erect for at least several hours a day, aided by a tilt or standing table. This activity reduces the frequency of urinary complications such as bladder infections due to stasis and lessens the degree of osteoporosis (bone loss) resulting from disuse.

Wheelchairs sometimes provide the benefits of community travel to the home-only walker. Power wheelchairs are available for children who have insufficient strength to manage a manual model. These chairs require a van and lift for transport because they do not fold. Scoliosis pads or other external spinal containment measures are almost always necessary by the time a child requires an electric wheelchair. Centered hand controls are desirable, again to prevent leaning in the chair. A portable electric, hydraulic, or mechanical lift facilitates the care of children who cannot transfer from chair to toilet or bed. A wheeled shower commode chair is desirable for transport from bathroom to bedroom. It may be placed directly over the toilet or rolled into an adapted shower stall. It may also be used at the bedside. Most such chairs are approximately 21 inches wide in order to fit through the average bathroom door.

SCOLIOSIS

In DMD spinal muscle weakness is symmetric and equal, and spinal curvature rarely occurs. When it does occur, it usually is accompanied by pelvic tilt resulting from uncorrected lower extremity contractures. Pelvic tilt unbalances the torso and causes the spine to curve to regain balance. Children who can stand and/or walk lock the joints in their low back, which inhibits scoliosis. This is one of the reasons why it is desirable to keep the DMD patient upright as long as possible. Therapeutic standing is an important part of the prophylactic treatment of these children even when they must use a wheelchair. The longer wheelchair use can be delayed, the less chance a child has of developing scoliosis when a wheelchair becomes necessary. This is especially true if spinal growth has been completed (approximately age 15 years in girls, 16 in boys) by the time the child finds full-time wheelchair use necessary.

After they start using a wheelchair, well over half of all children develop some degree of scoliosis. This may progress slowly, at approximately 2 to 3 degrees of curve a month, until the adolescent growth spurt at approximately age 13 years, when spinal curves may undergo rapid progression.

Severe scoliosis may interfere with breathing. Forced vital capacity—a measure of the amount of air that can be expelled forcibly from the lungs from a position of full inspiration—is decreased by approximately 4 percent for each 10 degrees of curve in the thorax (chest) and by the same amount for each year of age after onset of the curve. Scoliosis seldom occurs in the child who is upright and walking, but it frequently becomes a problem when he requires a wheelchair. As scoliosis progresses, the child needs to use his upper limbs for support because of impaired sitting balance. With an advanced curve there may be loss of functional head positioning and a distorted body image. Pain may accompany advancing deformity. For all these reasons, it is imperative that scoliosis be treated vigorously.

The tug of gravity on the spine may be relieved by periodically tilting the child back in his wheelchair. Lightweight plastic spinal braces sometimes are indicated for short-term daytime use to maintain upright sitting balance when curves measure less than 30 degrees. Specialized seating systems may serve the same purpose. Both the braces and the seating systems increase *lumbar lordosis* (swayback) in an effort to lock the joints of the lower spine, which inhibits scoliosis. It must be emphasized that these methods seldom *prevent* scoliosis. Rather, they *delay* the development of spinal deformity and reduce its rate of progression. At the same time, they may provide comfortable, functional seating.

Obesity contributes to scoliosis. A thin child who is kept well-balanced in his wheelchair has a better chance of developing a naturally stiff, straight spine than an obese child who sits slumped in the chair because his excess weight prevents proper sitting posture (Figure 6-2).

Spinal curves that are greater than 30 degrees and unstable usually require surgery. Such an operation can only be performed if the vital capacity (respiratory function) is within 30 percent to 40 percent of predicted normal and the child retains the ability to cough. The surgery, called *spinal fusion,* involves straightening curved segments of the spine and fixing them with metallic instrumentation augmented by bone graft. The result is a significant correction of the spinal curve, with a rigid spine in that segment of the spinal column that had been deformed. Spinal func-

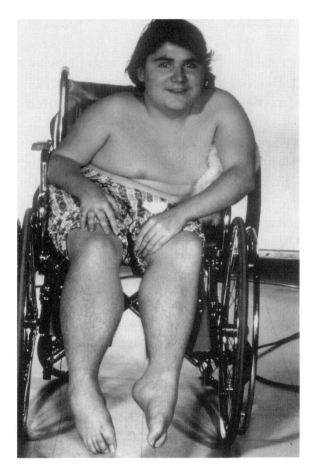

FIGURE 6–2 It is important to minimize obesity if a child is to avoid the development of scoliosis.

tion is maintained. The child will be able to sit upright in his chair and will be able to bend almost as well as he did before surgery. The arms are no longer needed to support the trunk and are freed for functional tasks. A spinal brace or other back support is not necessary after surgery. Recovery usually is rapid and without complication. However, in rare cases correcting the scoliosis may worsen breathing or swallowing.

The operation should be performed by a spinal surgeon (usually an orthopaedic surgeon) who is familiar with the problems of the DMD patient and is experienced in the procedure. It is equally important that the anesthesiologist be familiar with the problems of managing a patient with compromised respiratory function through a long surgical procedure. It goes without saying that the hospital should have state-of-the-art recovery, postoperative supportive, and rehabilitation facilities.

OBESITY

Dietary management is important throughout the course of muscular dystrophy, particularly after a child requires the use of a wheelchair. In contrast to a normal boy whose greatest weight increment occurs between 12 and 16 years, the child with DMD experiences his greatest weight gain between 10 and 13 years of age. Nutrition education should be provided to parents and patients, including an understanding of the four basic food groups—milk, meat, fruit/vegetable, grain, and the need to avoid too much fat, saturated fat, cholesterol, sugar, and salt (Figure 6-3). Adequate vitamin and mineral consumption should be stressed (this may require supplementation), and fiber and fluid intake should be emphasized.

Obesity occurs particularly after a wheelchair becomes necessary and hastens functional disability. Many children handle their anxiety by excessive eating, and well-meaning but ignorant caregivers often handle theirs by excessive feeding. It is easier to pre-

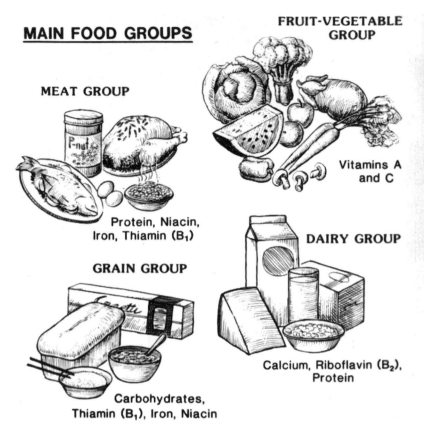

MAIN FOOD GROUPS

FRUIT-VEGETABLE GROUP

MEAT GROUP

Vitamins A and C

Protein, Niacin, Iron, Thiamin (B₁)

DAIRY GROUP

GRAIN GROUP

Calcium, Riboflavin (B₂), Protein

Carbohydrates, Thiamin (B₁), Iron, Niacin

FIGURE 6–3 Foods required for nutritional balance.

vent this complication than to treat it. The obese child should be provided a well-balanced, vitamin-supplemented diet of no less than 1200 calories. Children should be encouraged to choose fruits and vegetables as alternatives to high-calorie snacks. High-fiber foods and fruit juices aid in maintaining normal elimination. Only small amounts of milk products should be offered because of their mucus-producing tendency, which may interfere with respiration. Nondairy liquids and frozen products or lactose-free nonfat milk may be substituted. Wheelchair users often reduce

fluid intake and retain urine as long as possible
because they are reluctant to ask for toileting assistance. This may predispose the child to infection. Male
wheelchair users sometimes may benefit from the use
of a condom catheter urinary drainage system. In
addition to ensuring adequate fluid intake, foods such
as cereals, meats, poultry, fish, and cranberry juice,
which increase urinary acidity, are advised.

CONSTIPATION AND DIARRHEA

Because of inactivity, children who require wheelchairs
often develop constipation as the result of problems
with gastrointestinal transit time or other gastrointestinal dysfunction, decreased fluid and fiber intake
(use of low-fiber, highly refined foods), poor meal pat-
terning, and poor toileting habits. This problem should
be treated with natural means through the ingestion of
whole grain cereals, fresh vegetables (puréed), and
foods high in fiber. Fluid intake should be increased
and natural laxatives, such as prunes and stewed
fruits, should be taken with each meal. Meal patterns
should be regulated and the child should be encouraged
to respond to the urge to evacuate. Stool softeners and
morning suppositories sometimes are necessary. An
occasional enema (tap water, salt water, soap suds)
may be necessary, but excessive use may lead to fluid
and electrolyte imbalance and should be avoided. A pro-
fessional dietitian may help you with this and other
dietary-nutritional problems. A dietary consultation
may be arranged through your MDA clinic.

Diarrhea may be due to fecal impaction, lactase deficiency, laxative abuse, or the ingestion of certain

antacids. Treatment involves removing the cause and providing an antidiarrheal pill. Many medications alter the absorption and/or metabolism of nutrients and minerals. Mineral oil should not be used as a laxative because it affects the absorption of vitamins A, D, and K. Phenobarbital or Dilantin, which are prescribed as anticonvulsants, may decrease the absorption of calcium. Many antacids inhibit the absorption of phosphates.

OTHER PROBLEMS OF WHEELCHAIR USERS

If the child's legs are held in the "dependent" (down) position throughout the day, there may be reduction of circulation to the lower extremities, with edema (swelling) of the feet and ankles. This can be managed by frequent elevation of the legs, gentle massage from the toes toward the heart, and the use of lightweight elastic hosiery. For severe swelling, an externally applied pump in the form of plastic leggings called a sequential pressure device may be obtained through an OT or PT service.

Increased weakness and contracture always occurs and includes the upper extremities. The physical therapist can supervise a program of active and passive exercises for the arms and hands. Pressure pain in the buttocks resulting from long periods of seated immobility may be a problem. This can be treated by using a proper seat cushion. Several types are available, such as the Jay-cushion®, Roho pad®, eggcrate foam, Silastic™ padding, and so on. Seating specialists are available for consultation through your MDA clinic.

Sometimes spasm of a small muscle called the piriformis, which lies deep in the buttocks, may press on the

sciatic nerve. This causes sciatica, just like that resulting from a slipped disc in the back. This "piriformis syndrome" may be relieved by an injection of cortisone.

OCCUPATIONAL THERAPY

Occupational therapy is very important at this stage.
Particular attention should be paid to range of motion
exercises for the arms and hands to aid the ability to
use the upper extremities away from the body. Hand
and wrist splints may be indicated. Assistive devices,
such as reachers, eating aids, and adaptive clothing,
will increasingly be needed.

The occupational therapist should visit the home
to assess the need for architectural modifications (e.g.,
ramps, installed lifts) or other specialized equipment.
Architectural barriers in the school and community at
large should be similarly evaluated. A full-time atten-
dant at school often is necessary. Both PT and OT
emphasis at this time are on the performance of small
motor tasks, including what are termed *activities of
daily living* (ADLs), such as hygiene, eating, using
computers, and recreational activities.

INCREASED DEFORMITY

Foot and ankle deformity may continue to occur even
in a wheelchair-using child. Because of progressive
weakening and muscle imbalance, the foot and ankle
progressively turn in, leading to a so-called *inversion*
(inward twisting) at the ankle. This deformity is
inhibited, but not prevented, by wearing a brace. It

sometimes is seen in children who are still walking, in whom it may temporarily respond to stretching and heel-control shoe inserts. In the wheelchair user, the inversion deformity sometimes may progress to the point where it is painful. The twisted position of the feet prevents the use of normal footwear. Children should be encouraged to keep their feet well-positioned on the wheelchair footrests to inhibit the development of this malrotation.

Surgical correction is available either by releasing tight tendons and other soft tissues or by operating on the bones of the foot, during which appropriate wedges of bone are removed to correct the deformity.

QUESTIONS

Q: Do patients ever have problems with perineal (genital) hygiene and skin care when they require a wheelchair?

A: If the muscles of the hip become severely contracted, it may be difficult to provide perineal hygiene. This is one reason to continue hip stretching even when using a wheelchair. Patients seldom develop pressure ulcers from prolonged sitting because skin sensation remains intact. If a pressure ulcer does occur, it can be treated with an appropriate salve and dressing. Wheeled commode chairs with C- or W-shaped cushions allow access to the perineal area. Bidet equipment with warm water wash and warm air dry also are available.

Flaking of the skin around the hairline (seborrheic dermatitis, or dandruff) may occur, as may vascular reddening of the skin. The dandruff may be treated with any of a variety of proprietary products available at your local drugstore. The vascular reddening of the skin is not serious and does not require treatment.

Q: Are there any speech difficulties in Duchenne muscular dystrophy?

A: In advanced DMD there sometimes is enlargement of the tongue as well as a decreased rate of tongue and jaw movement. There also is weakness of the muscles of the mandible, which may lead to a thin vocal quality with excessive nasality when speaking. Impairment in the laryngeal muscles makes it difficult to cough, clear the throat, or sustain speaking. Respiratory muscle weakness may result in diminished vocal intensity. The child may have an enlarged tongue, which may protrude because there is a tendency to hold the mouth open. Consultation with a speech therapist for evaluation and treatment is recommended.

Q: Do wheelchair users undergo severe mental depression?

A: Children who are confined with almost complete lack of mobility sometimes suffer mental and emotional problems. Providing an environment in which independence is stressed and mobility is encouraged and enhanced, both at home and in the community, tends to allay such problems. A child who cannot propel a manual wheelchair is significantly empowered when provided with a power chair.

Q: Can using a cane or a walker help a child continue to ambulate independently?

A: Usually not, because these walking aids require upper extremity strength, which may be lacking. They also inhibit the postural adjustments necessary to maintain balance. However, walkers sometimes are used as standing aids and allow the occasional patient to take a few steps.

Q: Is there any test to determine bone age?

A: Yes. X-rays of the wrist are taken and degree of closure of the growth plates is compared with that normally found for each period of growth. It sometimes is important to know a child's bone age in deciding when to perform a spinal fusion.

Q: Is spinal fusion ever performed in a child who is still walking?

A: Occasionally in some of the more benign neuromuscular diseases, seldom if ever in DMD, because fusing the spine inhibits the postural upper torso shift required to balance and walk. For this reason a rigid torso brace (thoracolumbosacral orthosis, or TLSO) seldom is prescribed for a walking patient.

Q: What are some things the school can do to assist a student with DMD to adapt more easily?

A: A teacher may allow a student to leave classes early to get to his next class on time. The student could be allowed extra time to take tests. When prolonged writing is a problem, he could be allowed to use a tape recorder in class. Adapted computers allow some students full access to information and enhance the ability to respond. Where possible, all classes should be arranged on the same floor. If an elevator is available in the building, the student could be given permission to use it to go from class to class on different floors.

Q: Why is high school such a challenge to children with DMD?

A: High school is a challenge to every student, normal and otherwise. The school situation is much more complex than in grade school. The student has to move from classroom to classroom and interact with many teachers. The pace of academic work usually accelerates, with a heavier workload and more deadlines. The student with motor difficulties may have problems moving quickly through crowded hallways around a large school building.

Q: What can be done about architectural barriers in the community?

A: One can agitate against them by joining equal access groups, signing petitions, and writing letters to members of local and national governing bodies. Access to all public buildings is mandated by the Americans with Disabilities Act (ADA). Private schools may not be covered but may be interested in being "good citizens" for the special child.

Q: What about legal rights, access to health care, disability employment, and the like?

A: Local, city, state, and federal offices provide information about the legal rights of people with disabilities through employment, health care, and social and rehabilitation services. Your MDA program services coordinator can assist you in obtaining this information. This may be as simple as applying for a handicapped parking sticker or as complicated as filing for social security disability insurance.

Q: How do we handle questions about sex in a disabled adolescent?

A: In the same way that you would handle such questions if the child were not disabled. It is important to realize that sexual feelings, drives, and concerns are not affected in muscular dystrophy. Socializing with groups of friends of both sexes should be encouraged. Summer camps sponsored by MDA facilitate this. Dating should neither be pushed nor discouraged. It is up to the child to make this decision, whatever his age. Matters such as this require much patience and understanding. Sexual needs must be recognized and accepted, and the home should provide appropriate role models, privacy, and opportunity for learning. This involves open and frank discussion of all matters that affect the child, sexual or nonsexual.

Q: Is hand function impaired in muscular dystrophy?

A: In distal muscular dystrophy and myotonic muscular dystrophy, the muscles of the hands are involved early on. The hands may weaken late in the course of DMD. Shoulder, elbow, wrist, and finger contractures occur, usually after wheelchair confinement. These joints, like those in the legs, can be passively stretched to impede contractures, and splints are available to assist hand function.

7

LATE-LATE PROBLEMS

Eating difficulties are seldom seen in early DMD. When they occur, it usually is late in the disease. Dental malocclusion is common and may contribute to the inability to chew well. The esophagus is made up of voluntary (striated) muscle in its upper third, but involuntary (smooth) muscle also may be involved in DMD (Figure 7-1). Problems with swallowing are best assessed by *videofluoroscopy,* a modified barium swallowing study. Eating difficulties may arise from the following (see also Figure 7-2):

Eating difficulty due to feeding technique

1. Decreased ability to suck
   A. Treat by spooning food.
2. Weak grasp with inability to bring food to mouth
   A. Treat through the use of long eating implements, balanced forearm orthoses, and other feeding aids.

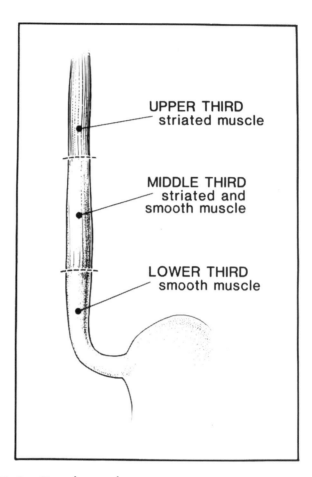

UPPER THIRD
striated muscle

MIDDLE THIRD
striated and
smooth muscle

LOWER THIRD
smooth muscle

FIGURE 7–1   Esophageal anatomy.

3. Improperly prepared food
   A. Treat by providing softened, puréed, or liquid foods.

Eating difficulty due to muscular weakness

1. Chewing weakness
   A. Treat with foods that require less vigorous chewing.

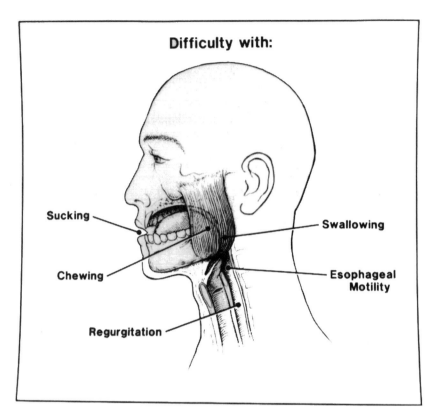

Difficulty with:

Sucking

Chewing

Regurgitation

Swallowing

Esophageal Motility

FIGURE 7–2   Causes of feeding disability.

2. Palatal weakness
    A. Thicker liquids are easier to swallow than thin ones. A patient with palatal weakness may swallow a malted milk easier than a glass of water.
3. Problems with motility of the GI tract. Dysfunction of involuntary muscle has been found in Duchenne muscular dystrophy. The following gastrointestinal problems have been reported.
    A. Weakness in the pharynx

    1. Increased possibility for aspiration of food
        a. Treat with instruction in proper position-
            ing (head and neck flexed forward, not
            back) to assist gravity by straightening
            the esophagus. Tube feedings.
  B. Esophageal weakness
    1. Regurgitation of food
        a. Treat with instruction in eating slowly,
            introducing soft and puréed foods into the
            diet, sitting upright for a time after
            meals, avoiding excessive fluids with
            meals, not eating a heavy meal close to
            bedtime, sleeping in a propped-up posi-
            tion. Atropine-like drugs may also help.
  C. Weakness of stomach muscles
    1. Stomach distention
        a. Treat with abdominal binder.
  D. Weakness of small bowel
    1. Obstruction or malabsorption
  E. Weakness of colon
    1. Dilatation of colon
  F. Gallbladder
    1. Decreased gallbladder contractility with an
        increased incidence of gallstones

D, E, and F require the attention of a pediatric gas-
troenterologist.

BREATHING

The *diaphragm* is a respiratory muscle that lies under
the lungs and separates the thorax from the abdomen.
It normally moves up and down when we breathe. The

lungs convey excess mucus and inhaled particles toward the mouth, where they can be coughed out. In advanced DMD, respiratory muscle weakness prevents this lung "housekeeping." Weakness of the abdominal muscles prevents adequate coughing. Obesity may contribute to breathing difficulty because more weight means more work for the muscles of respiration. Sedatives and cough suppressants should be avoided, particularly at night.

Sitting up, even during sleep, may make breathing and swallowing easier. The rental or purchase of a hospital bed can be arranged through your local MDA office, which will be able to offer guidance on the services and equipment that are most reliable and cost-effective. Equipment does not always have to be purchased; it sometimes may be rented or borrowed from the MDA equipment pool.

Breathing becomes more difficult as respiratory muscles weaken. This is a particular problem at night because the abdomen pushes up against the diaphragm when a person lies down. The patient who has difficulty with nighttime breathing may complain of nonrestorative sleep with fatigue on awakening, headaches, night sweats, nightmares, and an inability to get enough air if awakened at night. Other symptoms of lung underventilation include shortness of breath, daytime drowsiness, dysphagia (difficulty swallowing), poor concentration, anxiety, memory impairment, and decreased appetite. A thorough respiratory examination, sometimes including a sleep study (polysomnography), may clarify the nature and extent of respiratory disability and determine appropriate treatment. Vital capacity (the volume of air expelled after a deep breath) should be measured lying down. Blood level of oxygen can also be monitored by a fingerheld device called an oximeter. The ability to cough can also be assessed.

Children with DMD increasingly breathe with the diaphragm as chest muscles weaken and atrophy. It is important to realize that these children have essentially normal lungs; they just do not have enough muscle strength to breathe and cough. Administering oxygen will only suppress the body's natural drive to breathe. What is required instead is a program of noninvasive respiratory muscle treatments and aids to increase lung ventilation and cough flow. This therapy should be performed under the direction of a pulmonologist who is familiar with the respiratory problems of patients with neuromuscular disease and may include such measures as glossopharyngeal (frog) breathing, in which air is gulped and "stacked" until enough air enters the lungs for a normal breath volume, as well as the use of any of a variety of mechanical body ventilators that provide either negative or positive pressure to assist breathing. "Cough machines" also are available to help the patient cough. These therapies can significantly delay (even sometimes avoid) the need for more invasive measures to support respiration. Aids for nighttime breathing include measures such as continuous positive airway pressure (CPAP) and BiPAP, which provide oxygen under pressure on a timed cycle through assisted breathing with a fitted mask worn at night. CPAP delivers air at a constant pressure. The BiPAP machine delivers air at two pressures, one for inspiration and the other for expiration. These treatments rest the muscles of breathing so that the child will feel more rested and have more energy during the day.

When assistive ventilation is no longer satisfactory to maintain respiration, a tracheostomy may be required, in which a permanent breathing tube is placed at the base of the neck into the windpipe. This often is performed with sedation under local anesthesia. A ventilator may be attached to the tube to provide a constant source of oxygen. Such a ventilator or tank of oxygen is placed at the bedside or may be mounted on a motorized wheelchair. Children with tracheostomies who are on ventilators part- or full-time require special attention. Nonetheless, they are able to function comfortably in their wheelchairs with assisted ventilation. Modern tracheostomy tubes have valves that permit near-normal conversation. Although special caretaking is necessary (sometimes round-the-clock care), the quality of life of these patients is considerably enhanced by assisting their breathing.

Weakness in swallowing may result in sucking liquid or food into the lungs instead of into the esophagus. This is called *aspiration* and may cause pneumonia. In severe cases the child must be tube-fed. A gastrostomy tube inserted directly into the stomach may prevent this. In this procedure (percutaneous endoscopic gastrostomy, or PEG), an opening is established from the skin to the stomach. This usually can be done under local anesthesia. Liquid nutriments are delivered through the tube into the stomach. This bypasses the mouth and throat, eliminating any chance of choking or aspiration. An adequate fiber and caloric level, as defined and adjusted by a dietitian, may be maintained through tube feeding. Often nutritionally balanced liquid food such as Ensure® or Jevity® is used.

CARDIAC PROBLEMS

Disability from cardiomyopathy may be masked or seem insignificant compared with that imposed by other muscle weakness in advanced DMD. However, the heart may fail because of respiratory difficulties. This condition, which is called *cor pulmonale,* results from right heart strain because of trouble with breathing. Consultation with a cardiologist who is familiar with the problem of involvement of the heart muscle is advised. Cardiac failure is unusual because very little stress is placed on the heart. Treatment of arrhythmia (irregular rhythm) or other cardiac problems is the same as that for any patient who has a similar cardiac problem.

QUESTIONS

Q: Why is it important to maintain some motion in the hips even in the patient who uses a wheelchair?

A: For ease of transfer and comfort. Also, perineal care is facilitated. In young women the incidence of vaginal infections is increased when perineal hygiene is a problem. Baby wipes are easy to use for this. There also are toilet attachments that provide the features of a bidet with a warm water wash and air dry.

Q: Are over-the-counter laxatives a good treatment for severe constipation in the wheelchair patient?

A: As long as they are not taken on a regular basis. Bowel habits differ in these children. Some have a bowel movement every day, some every several days, and some only about once a week. As long as the patient is not uncomfortable, there is no need for concern. However, weakness of the muscles of the abdomen makes it difficult to evacuate the bowel properly and sometimes a fecal impaction may occur. This often has to be manually removed by a physician or nurse.

Q: My son wakes up frequently at night asking to be turned. Is there any way to keep him comfortable so that we can all get a good night's rest?

A: Everyone normally changes position frequently during sleep to relieve skin pressure. The child weakened by muscular dystrophy is unable to move enough to relieve himself in this way. A firm mattress usually is recommended but some children are more comfortable sleeping on a firm waterbed or air mattress. Using a pillow between the legs and pillows to cushion and support the child is helpful. Nylon or satin sheets and/or pajamas decrease friction and facilitate moving in bed. Electric blankets or lightweight comforters are warm and lighter than the ordinary blanket. Over-bed foot cradles may be beneficial. These keep the covers off the child's legs for comfort, enabling him to move freely in bed without fighting the weight of blankets. Special cushions made of foam or other synthetic materials may be helpful. Special mattresses that employ alternating pressure pads may prevent skin discomfort and decrease the number of times a patient requires turning at night.

Q: Why are upper respiratory tract infections such a threat in the DMD child, particularly when using a wheelchair?

A: Because of decreased pulmonary function and poor respiratory toilet, they may lead to a more serious infection, bronchitis, and even pneumonia. It is important to keep the child well-hydrated by drinking liquids frequently during the day and to treat any respiratory infection vigorously with appropriate antibiotics and supportive care. It may be necessary to have more aggressive respiratory therapy, including positioning for postural drainage, education in diaphragmatic breathing, chest therapy, and to use equipment such as an incentive spirometer or even a portable intermittent positive pressure breathing (IPPB) apparatus. Evaluation and specific treatment can be arranged through consultation with a pulmonary therapist.

Q: What are some things to think about when considering a tracheostomy?

A: Some youngsters and their families decide that, when indicated, tracheostomy with permanent ventilatory support is a viable choice for a prolonged life with increased quality of living. Such a decision should be made thoughtfully, with consideration given to all aspects of this important choice, including the considerable care and not inconsiderable cost of the 24-hour nursing attention sometimes necessary for maintenance. Discussion with your MDA clinic team will help you explore your options and understand what this might mean to the child and his family. In any case, the decision of whether to perform a tracheostomy should be made electively before it becomes a medical crisis that requires a hasty and often poorly examined choice.

Q: What assistive devices can provide control for those people requiring a wheelchair who lack strength in their hands to perform tasks or even work a motorized chair?

A: There are many. Some examples are wheelchair-mounted robotic arms for eating; chin, tongue, and sip-and-puff wheelchair controls; and—although not exactly a "device"—service dogs that can operate switches, open doors, and obtain help if needed.

Q: What types of mechanical ventilation systems do not require nasal tubes or mouthpieces?

A: The "pneumobelt" uses an inflatable abdominal sack that applies pressure, pushing air out of the lungs. When it deflates, gravity pulls the abdominal contents down, pulling air back in. The "rocking bed" tips the head of the bed down to deflate the lungs and tips the foot down to reinflate. The cuirass (shell ventilator) straps over the chest and upper abdomen. Evacuation of the rigid shell inflates the lungs, and repressuring it deflates them.

Q: The burden of taking care of a severely ill adolescent who must use a wheelchair is sometimes overwhelming. I don't seem to have enough time or energy to cope with the ever-present urgent demands. What can I do about this?

A: In muscular dystrophy the family is the patient. Caregivers have to care for themselves if they are going to continue helping their loved one to the best of their ability. It is important to arrange to give yourself a break by having a trained person take over your duties for a time. It also is important for you to understand the emotional aspect of the situation, including your own feelings. This usually requires counseling. Some MDA clinics have parent support groups that allow parents to share feelings, concerns, and ideas about coping with the changes in their lives and the lives of their children.

Q: How do we access resources for the care of our child with DMD?

A: Educational booklets as well as lists of books and information regarding medical equipment, financial, legal and medical resources, websites and forums, research, and other information are all available through the Muscular Dystrophy Association, 3300 E. Sunrise Drive, Tucson, Arizona 85718, phone 800/572-1717, WWW.MDAUSA.ORG, or your local MDA office.

Q: What types of help are available for home care of the child with muscular dystrophy?

A: Everything from babysitting and respite care to in-home nursing or home care agencies to hospice home services for a person with advanced DMD. Your MDA patient service coordinator or social worker can assist you in making appropriate arrangements.

8

A CAREGIVER'S SELF-HELP GUIDE

Caring for someone with muscular dystrophy requires constant adaptation to a changing situation. Much time and energy is required, priorities have to be shuffled, and powerful emotions are involved. In the face of these problems, it is only normal to feel inadequate from time to time. This can border on depression, and caregiver burnout is frequently seen. Help for this is available. There are books, organizations, and computer web pages to help you face the stress engendered by the task of caregiving.

But first you have to take charge of your own health. You cannot help anyone else if you break down physically or emotionally. You must make time for yourself, and this may involve delegating tasks to family and friends. Sometimes it is necessary to hire a trained health care worker. You must learn to ask for help.

You have to get in the habit of creating a space where you can periodically back off and relax. You will find that changes in the dynamics of your family, accompanied by significant loss of leisure and feelings of isolation, can lead to depression. This can also be a test for your marriage. Because of their work routines, fathers tend to be less disrupted by the presence of a seriously ill, home-bound child than are mothers. Demands on the mother's time and strength are severe. Neighbors are not always tactful, and strangers provoke self-consciousness and shame. It is not only important—it is vital that you find time to spend with your spouse and that you continue to keep lines of communication open. Expressing fear, frustration, anger, and the other emotions engendered in this situation helps to relieve these feelings. Changing your expectations and redefining individual and family goals make coping less frustrating.

ESPECIALLY FOR PARENTS

Learning that your child has a serious illness is a tremendous blow to parents. Many describe the event as a "knife stuck in the heart," "the end of the world," "a black cloud descending over us," and similar responses that indicate depression and despair. Common reactions to this situation include denial, which rapidly merges with anger. Anger can impede communication between parents. Early on, the anger can be so intense that it involves almost anyone because it is triggered by feelings of grief and inexplicable loss that one does not know how to explain or deal with.

Another reaction is fear. This is mostly fear of the unknown. Parents wonder what will happen to their child as he matures. "Will he have enough strength to go to school?" "Will he be capable of getting married and having a family of his own?" The first thoughts that parents have upon receiving the diagnosis of muscular dystrophy are usually very bleak. They expect the worst. They wonder how their family will be affected. There are many unknowns. These include the fear of rejection by society and concern about how they will react to their child as time goes by.

Feelings of guilt also play a role. Parents ask themselves whether they had a part in causing the disease. Much remorse can be avoided by recognizing the genetic causes of the child's disability. Many parents express spiritual interpretations of blame and punishment. "Why has God seen fit to do this to me now?" is a commonly asked question. This traumatic period is marked by confusion as a result of not fully understanding what is happening and what will happen. Parents have difficulty making sense of the information they are receiving. They feel powerless to change what is happening. They want to feel competent, yet they must rely on information provided by strangers to whom they have not yet bonded. Their value system, and indeed their very egos, are threatened by the disappointment that their child is defective. They may experience rejection of the child by other family members or even medical personnel. A not uncommon form of rejection is a parental "death wish" for the child. Many parents report this at their deepest point of depression. Many things can be done to help a parent through this period of trauma. There are constructive actions to be taken and there are sources of help, communication, and reassurance.

One thing a parent can do is seek the assistance of another parent of a child with muscular dystrophy or a group of such parents. In this way, the almost universal feeling of isolation at the time of diagnosis is eased. Recognizing that you are not alone may diminish the flood of strong emotions that inevitably accompany the diagnosis of muscular dystrophy. Feelings of separateness and isolation can be diminished by realizing that they have been experienced by many others and that understanding and constructive help are available to you and your child.

Communication of feelings with a mate may increase a couple's collective strength. You can also talk to your other children and be aware of their needs. The temptation may be to close up emotionally, but talking with a significant other in your life—best friend, parent, clergyman, or counselor when warranted—goes a long way toward easing the emotional burden. Pain shared is not nearly as hard to bear as is pain in isolation. It is good to have a philosophy of living one day at a time. Fear of the future is immobilizing. Living with the reality and challenges of each day is much more manageable. Life satisfaction of a disabled child focuses on social relationships, reorganization of goals, and his or her immediate environment. These things can be effected by parental enterprise.

Learning medical terminology is important. Parents and caretakers should be constantly seeking information. A good method is to list questions before appointments and to keep copies of all written documentation from teachers, physicians, and therapists. In that way, you will be less intimidated by medical encounters. There is no shame in showing emotion. Fathers in particular may think it is a sign of weakness to let people know how badly they feel. They should understand that revealing feelings does not diminish one's strength. Adopting a grateful attitude for any positive things in your life, of which there may be many, can help you learn to deal with bitterness and anger and help you maintain a positive outlook.

Accepting life the way it is means to stay in touch with reality. There are some things that we must recognize and change and other things that we cannot change. There are many things that can be changed in the management of a child with muscular dystrophy. The task for parents is to set about making these changes. With current research accelerating to find a cure for muscular dystrophy, time may be on the side of many parents with newly diagnosed children. Assistance is available to help you with whatever problems you are having with your child. Contacting the proper sources can help you find such support. In the meantime, you must take care of yourself, avoiding pity, but developing empathy toward your child and those with whom he comes in contact. This will help you from becoming unduly judgmental and expending energy being concerned over those who do not respond toward your child or situation in ways that you might prefer. Try to keep your daily routines as normal as possible, remembering that this is your child and that even though he or she is different from other children, he is no less valuable, less human, less important, or less in need of your love and parenting. Love and enjoy your child as a child first and a disabled child second.

RESEARCH

9

WHAT THE FUTURE HOLDS

Only a few years ago we had little idea as to the definitive cause of Duchenne muscular dystrophy and related neuromuscular conditions. At that time there was no promise of a cure. This has all changed. Since the discovery of the dystrophin gene in 1986, scientists have been actively engaged in gene therapy research in an effort to develop a genetically engineered treatment for Duchenne muscular dystrophy. To date, muscle genes have been isolated and successfully used in animal models. It is apparent that muscular dystrophy *can* be medically managed; it is only a question of *when* this will be accomplished.

The dedicated and elegant work of investigators in this field has developed a highly altered version of an adenovirus (cold virus). All viral DNA (genetic material) was removed from this virus, which opened up enough space to accommodate the dystrophin gene. Also, removal of its viral genes prevents the virus from triggering an immune response after it gets into muscle. Other viral *vectors* (transporters) are currently being investigated. One is the adeno-associated virus, a small virus that does not cause any disease. Adeno-associated virus spreads well throughout muscle fibers, inserting the gene with stability. It does not evoke an immune response and persists in expressing the inserted gene for a long time. Similar results with these viruses have been documented in neurons (nerve cells).

It has been shown that DNA alone ("naked DNA") can be forced (under pressure with nearby blood vessels tied off) into muscle fibers, where it remains and functions. This opens the possibility of intraarterial delivery of genes.

Clinical research is currently being conducted at several academic sites. These studies involve injecting a series of boys with Duchenne muscular dystrophy with virus that has been packed with a normal dystrophin gene, carrying instructions for the protein that their muscles lack. The success of this research program will have implications as well for the treatment of both Becker and limb-girdle muscular dystrophy, indeed for the management of any neuromuscular disease whose origin lies in a defect of the genetic material. Unfortunately, little effect can be expected in advanced disease because there so far is no way to regenerate severely damaged muscle.

Other lines of investigation include increasing the synthesis or "up-regulation" of compensatory proteins when the protein dystrophin is deficient. One of these is the muscle protein *utrophin,* which normally is located at the junction between nerves and muscles.

New molecular technologies are taking a long hard look at this possibility. Yet another intriguing idea is the manipulation of *telomerase,* a cellular enzyme that controls growth, to grow muscle cells that can replace those depleted in muscular dystrophy. *Myostatin* is a muscle protein that plays a key role in the regulation of muscle growth and development. When the myostatin gene is inactivated, muscle undergoes extensive changes characterized by muscle hypertrophy (muscle fiber enlargement) and hyperplasia (an increase in the number of muscle fibers). It appears that myostatin is a regulatory molecule in the pathway that controls the maturation of muscle. Research into its inhibition may prove valuable in the stimulation of muscle growth and replacement.

The role of certain "growth factors," as well as calcium-regulating drugs and other critical processes, enzymes, and metabolites in muscle, is being vigorously pursued by MDA-sponsored scientists.

Aggressive therapy-oriented research continues to be conducted with methods of treatment. Clinical trials of the steroid drugs prednisone and oxandrolone (in DMD) as well as the drug albuterol (in FSH dystrophy) are ongoing. All three drugs have shown promise in preserving muscle despite the presence of an underlying genetic abnormality. Drugs by design (synthesis) rather than discovery (in the natural state) hold promise for future treatments.

While researchers are searching for cures for neuromuscular diseases, others have been developing new systems of bracing in an effort to keep patients standing and walking as long as possible. Some of these experimental braces stimulate muscular response, whereas others constrain spasticity.

Special electrical stimulation of the muscles controlling the spine in an effort to inhibit scoliosis is under study. Comfortable yet supportive wheelchair seating systems using newly discovered fabrication techniques assist in the management of the neuromuscular patient's spine. New bracing techniques using a cable-loaded mechanism may provide a reciprocating gait in patients lacking lower extremity strength.

Many challenges remain, but as we learn more and more about these diseases continued research will undoubtedly open doors to treatment and cure.

In summary, incurable—for now—is not untreatable, and with patience and skill, incurable should soon become curable.

Appendix A

ROBERT'S STORY

Robert D. was the product of a normal full-term pregnancy. The family history was positive in that his first cousin, a son of his mother's sister, had a progressive debilitating neuromuscular disease. Robert did not kick much while he was carried in utero. His birth was normal but he walked late, complained of cramping in his legs on activity, and was considered a "clumsy child." Robert was of normal intelligence. He had increasing difficulty keeping up with other children during play. At age 4 years, he was seen by a physician who diagnosed "flat feet" and prescribed special shoes. Robert continued to show signs of weakness. He fell frequently and had difficulty ascending stairs and jumping. When rising from a seated position, he "climbed up himself." He had no bowel or bladder difficulty, nor did he have trouble breathing or swallowing. Although his walking gait was normal, he waddled when he ran.

At 5 years of age Robert was examined by a neurologist. His CK level was 20,000 (more than 100 times normal). Examination revealed symmetric weakness in his shoulders, hips, and knees. His deep tendon reflexes were depressed and his enlarged calves had a "rubbery" feel. He had modest contractures of his heel cords and tended to walk on his toes. There was no indication of the presence of an inflammatory myopathy. Electrical studies were not deemed necessary. DNA examination of Robert's blood failed to show a point mutation (deletion), so a muscle biopsy was obtained, which revealed an almost complete lack of dystrophin. The diagnosis of Duchenne muscular dystrophy was made and a Duchenne pedigree was confirmed by correspondence with the physician who had made a similar diagnosis on Robert's cousin.

Because Robert was somewhat overweight and had difficulty controlling his appetite, it was decided not to place him on steroids for the time being because they stimulate appetite. A physical therapist instructed Robert's parents in stretching exercises for his tight heel cords. An occupational therapist reviewed activities at home and at school that might help in his management. A dietitian provided a diet to reduce weight. A social worker was consulted concerning his adjustment at home and in the community and also contacted the school to inform them of the diagnosis and the fact that Robert would have difficulty managing stairs and required an adaptive physical education class.

If Robert can maintain his diet, he may be placed on steroids. In any case, he will continue to be seen on a regular basis. By the time he is 9 to 12 years of age, he might require tendon releases and bracing of his legs to continue standing and walking. A wheelchair may become necessary sometime in his teens. A spinal fusion could be indicated if he develops scoliosis. Treatment of cardiac and respiratory complications will be available if needed.

It is hoped that research will develop therapies to arrest Robert's disease or even allow him to recoup his strength.

Appendix B

SUGGESTIONS FOR FURTHER READING

There are many books that deal with neuromuscular disease—the object here is not to overwhelm you, so I have selected a few that can provide more specific information should you desire it.

BOOKLETS AVAILABLE FROM MDA

"Everybody's Different, Nobody's Perfect." Written for the child with muscular dystrophy

"Hey, I'm Here Too!" Written for normal siblings of the child with muscle disease

"101 Hints to 'Help-With-Ease' for Patients with Neuromuscular Disease." Handy ways to facilitate tasks of daily living at home and in the community

"A Teacher's Guide to Duchenne Muscular Dystrophy." Facts about muscular dystrophy for teachers and school personnel

"Breathe Easy: Respiratory Care for Children with Muscular Dystrophy"

"Journey of Love." A parents' guide to Duchenne muscular dystrophy. Excellent presentation of basic science, physical and emotional needs, education and the family. Extensive list of readings and resources

"Quest," bimonthly MDA magazine. Feature articles on neuromuscular disease. Covers current research

BOOKS

"The Resourceful Caregiver," helping family caregivers help themselves, by the National Family Caregivers Association, Mosby Lifeline (1996). Call 800-325-4177

"Muscle Disorders in Childhood," 2nd ed., V. Dubowitz, M.D., W.B. Saunders Co., London, Philadelphia, 1995. Standard textbook on the subject

"Muscle and Its Diseases," I.M. Siegel, Yearbook Medical Publishers, Inc., Chicago, London, 1986. An outline primer of basic science and clinical method which covers diagnosis, biomechanics, and treatment

"Duchenne Muscular Dystrophy," Alan E.H. Emery, Oxford Medical Publications, 1987. Focuses on DMD; excellent discussion of genetics of this disease

"Evaluation and Treatment of Myopathies," R. Griggs, M.D., J. Mendell, M.D., R. Miller, M.D., F.A. Davis Co., Philadelphia, 1995. Well-rounded, clearly written text, up-to-date methods of diagnosis and treatment

"Guide to the Evaluation and Management of Neuromuscular Disease," John R. Bach, M.D., Hanley & Belfus, Philadelphia, 1994. Excellent guide to evaluation and management, particularly of respiratory problems

"Myology (Basic and Clinical)," 2nd ed., A.G. Engel, M.D., C. Franzini-Armstrong, Ph.D. McGraw-Hill, Inc., N.Y., 1994. One of the most complete (2 volumes) and highly detailed texts available. Covers all aspects of muscle disease, basic science and clinical

Appendix C

GLOSSARY

Abduct—To draw away from the midline of a limb or the body

Abiotrophy—Progressive loss of tissue vitality found in a degenerative hereditary disease

Achilles tendon—Heel cord

Adduct—To draw toward the midline of a limb or the body.

Antibody—An immunoglobulin molecule that interacts only with the antigen that induces its synthesis or with antigen closely related to it

Antigen—Any substance that, under appropriate conditions, will induce a specific immune response and react with the products of that response

Atrophy—Wasting

Balance (vector)—The force line (vector) produced on weight bearing which should keep the body upright

Becker (muscular dystrophy)—A primary X-linked myopathy resulting from decrease or abnormality of dystrophin. Clinical presentation is similar to that of Duchenne dystrophy but onset usually is later and progress is slower.

Biarticular (muscles)—Muscles that span two joints, causing movement at each on contraction

Bioelectric (responses)—The electrical response that is generated by muscle and nerve tissue

Cardiomyopathy—Noninflammatory disease of the heart muscle

Carrier—A person who harbors a recessive gene and therefore does not usually manifest symptoms of the disease but may transmit the gene to off-spring

Congenital—Existing at, and usually before, birth

Creatine kinase (CK)—The enzyme that catalyzes the phosphorylation of creatine by ATP to form phosphocreatine

DAG—Dystrophin-associated glycoprotein—Membranous molecular protein construct associated with dystrophin

Deep tendon reflexes—Involuntary contraction of a muscle after brief stretching caused by percussion of its tendon. Some deep tendon reflexes are the triceps reflex, the biceps reflex, the patellar reflex, and the Achilles reflex.

Distal myopathy—A type of muscle disease in which the distal muscles (those of the hands and the feet) are primarily involved. Certain other myopathies may have distal weakness as part of their presentation.

Dominant trait—A genetic pedigree in which the defective gene is carried by one parent, who expresses the disease. Fifty percent of his or her offspring (irrespective of gender) are at risk for inheriting the disease.

Dysmorphic (features)—Malformed

Eccentric (contraction)—Contraction of a muscle while it is lengthening

Electrodiagnosis—Refers generally to electrical techniques such as electromyography (EMG) and nerve conduction velocity (NCV) studies

Emery-Dreifuss muscular dystrophy—An X-linked myopathy with insidious onset in childhood. Signature findings include severe contractures of the neck and spine. There is slow progression without loss of ambulation. By mid-adulthood, cardiac conduction defects occur, which may cause sudden death.

Enzyme—A protein catalyst that accelerates chemical reactions without itself being destroyed or altered

Erythrocyte sedimentation rate (ESR)—Rather nonspecific blood test for inflammation

Esophagus—Swallowing tube between pharynx (back of mouth) and stomach

Extend—To straighten

Fasciculation—Brief muscle twitching, usually visible through the skin, representing spontaneous discharge of muscle fibers, seen in neurogenic muscle atrophy

Flex—To bend

Floppy infant—Hypotonia seen at birth. May be present in a number of conditions, including congenital muscular dystrophy, morphologically specific myopathies, spinal muscular atrophy type I, brain and/or spinal cord damage or lesion, and so forth.

Foot drop—Weakness in the ability to dorsiflex (bring up) the foot at the ankle. This results in a "slapping" gait, dragging the foot and tripping on the toes.

Friedreich's ataxia—An autosomal recessive disease secondary to spinocerebellar degeneration and characterized by peripheral neuropathy with spastic paraplegia, ataxia, foot and spinal deformity, ocular changes, and mental deficiency

Gait analysis—Analysis of gait, usually on a computerized walkway monitored by television. The technique is useful, even essential, in pinpointing specific motor abnormalities so that therapy such as surgery and bracing can be planned with scientific exactitude.

Gastrocsoleus—The muscle complex of the gastrocnemius and the soleus, which comprise the major muscle bulk of the calf and activate the Achilles tendon

Gowers' (sign)—Inability to rise from the seated position without support by "climbing up" the legs, due to quadriceps muscle and hip extensor weakness resulting in inability to extend (straighten) these joints. Also called the "tripod" sign

Heel cord—The tendon of the triceps surae muscle group, which is composed of the medial and lateral heads of the gastrocnemius and the soleus muscle. The "Achilles" tendon. The strongest tendon in the body, it plantarflexes the foot for toe-off during gait.

HMSN—Hereditary motor and sensory neuropathy. Charcot-Marie-Tooth disease

Hyperkalemic (periodic paralysis)—A condition of paralysis accompanied by an elevated blood potassium level. Hypokalemic periodic paralysis, in which the level of blood potassium is lower than normal, and normokalemic paralysis also occur.

Hypertrophy—Enlargement of muscle such as occurs in the calves of children with Duchenne muscular dystrophy

Hypotonia—Reduction of muscle tone

Idiopathic—Of unknown causation (from the Greek *idios*—private)

Inborn metabolic error—Genetically determined biomechanical disorder in which an enzyme defect produces pathologic consequences at birth

Joint—An articulation between two or more bones of the skeleton that permits motion. Joints may be fibrous, cartilaginous, or synovial. Synovial joints are configured in different ways to provide a large variety of movements. Some synovial joints have a condyloid shape. Others are gliding, hinge, ball-and-socket, saddle, or pivot-shaped.

Kinesthetic—Related to the motion of the human body

Kyphoscoliosis—Both backward and lateral curvature of the spine

LGD—Limb-girdle dystrophy. A dystrophinopathy (dystrophin pathology) in which dystrophin is present but decreased or altered. Clinical presentation is akin to Duchenne muscular dystrophy, but of later onset and slower progression. Inheritance may be autosomal recessive or dominant.

Lordosis—The anterior concavity of the curvature of the lumbar (and cervical) spine when viewed from the side. Synonyms include hollow back, saddleback, and swayback. The opposite deformity is kyphosis.

Mitochondrial myopathy—Myopathy secondary to defect in mitochondrial metabolism

Morphologically specific myopathy—Congenital myopathy named for specific morphologic change found on microscopy. Some examples are central core disease, nemaline rod disease, and myotubular myopathy. These diseases have a similar clinical picture, which includes hypotonia after birth, slowly progressive generalized muscular weakness, normal CK, and dysmorphic skeletal features

Motor neuron disease—Amyotrophic lateral sclerosis (ALS, Lou Gehrig's disease)

Myositis—Inflammation of muscle

Myopathy—Disease of muscle

Myotonia congenita—Thomsen's disease, a congenital condition of muscular hypertrophy with stiffness and weakness; relieved by exercise

NCV (nerve conduction velocity)—The velocity at which electrical current is conducted along nerve. Slowed in hereditary sensory and motor neuropathy type I and other demyelinating disease

Newton's Third Law—Physical law stating that every force is countered by an equal and opposite force. Useful in analyzing gait patterns in neuromuscular disease

Occupational therapy—The medical specialty that trains and assists patients to attend to the tasks of daily living at home and in the workplace

Oculopharyngeal myopathy—A myopathy common in French-Canadian and Spanish-American families. Regarded as a mitochondrial disease and characterized by external ophthalmoplegia with dysphagia. Onset is in the third or fourth decade and pedigree usually is autosomal dominant

Ophthalmoplegia—Weakness of the eye muscles

Orthoses—New terminology for "braces"

Pes cavus—Elevated long arch of the foot; seen in Charcot-Marie-Tooth disease and other neuropathic conditions

Plasmapheresis—The removal of plasma from the blood with retransfusion of the formed elements plus normal plasma back into the donor

Prone—Lying face downward

Proprioception—Perception of body position mediated by proprioceptor organs found in muscles and tendons

Ptosis—Drooping of the upper eyelid

Quadriceps—The four-headed muscle of the front of the thigh which attaches to the patella (kneecap) and extends (straightens) the knee and flexes (bends) the hip

Recessive trait—Genetic trait incapable of expression unless the defective gene is carried by both parents whose children, regardless of gender, are at 25 percent risk of inheriting the trait

Regeneration—Attempt of diseased muscle to repair itself during cycle of degeneration-regeneration

Respiration—Breathing

Scale effect—First described by Galileo, tells us that for every unit linear increase in a solid body, the surface area of the body increases by the square of the unit, its volume by the unit cubed. This explains why a patient with even an inactive condition limiting his ultimate muscle mass may, although initially ambulatory, eventually lose the ability to walk with growth.

Scapular winging—Protrusion of the shoulder blades due to muscle weakness in facioscapulohumeral muscular dystrophy. This deformity inhibits shoulder movement

SCARMD—Severe-childhood-autosomal-recessive-muscular dystrophy—Duchenne-like muscular dystrophy found in either sex and due to a deficiency or abnormality of dystrophin-associated glycoprotein

Shark mouth—Inverted V configuration of the upper lip seen in congenital myotonic dystrophy

Single fiber EMG—Test of electrical activity of a single muscle fiber. Useful in diagnosis and research of certain neuromuscular conditions

Supine—Lying with the face upward

Tachycardia—Rapid heartbeat

Tachypnea—Rapid respiration

Talipes equinovarus—Club foot in which the foot is twisted down and in on the ankle

Tongue fasciculations—Abnormal twitching of the tongue (a skinned muscle) usually accompanied by atrophy and found in neuropathic conditions such as spinal muscular atrophy and ALS

Upper motor neuron (also called a motoneuron)—The upper motor neurons are those in the cerebral cortex that conduct impulses to the cranial nerves or the spinal cord. Upper motor neuron signs include limb spasticity.

Vasculitis—Inflammation of blood vessels

Vectorcardiography—The measurement, transmitted by electrocardiographic leads, of the display (usually on an oscilloscope) of the direction and magnitude (vector) of the electromotive heart forces during a complete cardiac cycle

Vertebral caninization—Increase in the relative height of the vertebral bodies, which may ultimately become square in shape, as in the quadruped, which is seen in children chronically bedridden for any cause as well as in Duchenne muscular dystrophy and other selected myopathies

Vital capacity—Respiratory capacity

Waddling gait—Duck-like ambulation seen in advancing Duchenne muscular dystrophy, due to weakness of hip musculature

Wedge osteotomy—Corrective orthopaedic operation in which wedges of bone are removed to produce a more normal shape and position of the foot or other body member

Work hypertrophy—Enlargement of muscles due to exercise. Seen in the calves of patients with Duchenne muscular dystrophy early in their disease

X (linked)—Hereditary pedigree where the defective gene is on the X (sex) chromosome. Maternal transmission is exclusively to male offspring (50 percent risk). Females are at 50 percent jeopardy of being carriers.

XO gonadal dysgenesis—Turner's syndrome. A genetic trait leading to female masculinization with expression of a disease that appears like Duchenne muscular dystrophy

Index